HORIZONS IN CANCER RESEARCH

HORIZONS IN CANCER RESEARCH

VOLUME 63

HORIZONS IN CANCER RESEARCH

Additional books in this series can be found on Nova's website
under the Series tab.

Additional e-books in this series can be found on Nova's website
under the eBook tab.

HORIZONS IN CANCER RESEARCH

HORIZONS IN CANCER RESEARCH

VOLUME 63

HIROTO S. WATANABE
EDITOR

New York

Library of Congress Cataloging-in-Publication Data

ISBN: 978-1-53610-013-6

ISSN: 2159-1326

Published by Nova Science Publishers, Inc. † New York

CONTENTS

PREFACE

This book presents original results on the leading edge of cancer research. Chapter One reviews the most recent advances in the management, analyses the best possible treatment in each scenario, and discusses the future research direction on brain metastases from non-small cell lung cancer. Chapter Two discusses the positive effects of microscopic complete resection on controlling the local recurrence of a single brain metastasis. Chapter Three encapsulates the trends of the computer-aided diagnosis (CAD) development for the estimation of tumor malignancy. Chapter Four examines dendritic cells cross talk with cytomegalovirus pp65-specific cytotoxic T cells, $V\gamma\ 9\gamma\ \delta$ T cells, and invariant NKT cells in patients with glioblastoma multiforme. Chapter Five addresses CD8+ T cell activation and regulation in the skin, paying special attention to what it is known about CD8+ T cell activity and its link with SCC development. Chapter Six discusses knowledge of the molecular basis of anti-cancer drug resistance and the mechanisms through which triterpenoids modulate ABC transporter-mediated multi drug resistance. Chapter Seven reviews cancer and heparan sulfate alterations. Chapter Eight focuses on *Ganoderma lucidum* targeting apoptosis. Chapter Nine examines the integrated model of cAMP-dependent DNA expression which reveals an inverse relationship between cancer and neurodegeneration. Chapter Ten studies the prognosis of male breast cancer.

Chapter 1 - Brain metastases (BMs) from NSCLC cause significant morbidity and mortality for patients and major challenge in the management and care. BMs with increasing incidence in the current era of targeted therapy and immunotherapy has become a more important clinical issue. This is because patients tend to live longer from more effective therapy. MRI or CT of the brain has been incorporated in the routine tests of staging newly diagnosed

NSCLC. Thus more asymptomatic BMs have been discovered. Therefore BMs have attracted a lot of attention from academic and private oncologists and the management has transformed to new paradigms. Whole brain radiation (WBRT) is no longer the standard therapy for BMs. Once the BMs are confirmed, treatment is often based on the presence of driver mutations of primary NSCLC mass and if the mutation is drugable or not. Tyrosine kinase inhibitor is usually used to treat NSCLC with a sensitive mutation. Stereotactic Radiation (SRS) has gradually replaced WBRT especially in patients with less than 10 metastatic lesions. Radiation as the first line therapy is often reserved for NSCLC patients without driver mutations. This chapter reviews the most recent advances in the management, analyses the best possible treatment in each scenario, and discusses the future research direction on BMs from NSCLC.

Chapter 2 - Background; The influence on therapeutic outcome of the wide surgical resection of brain metastasis (BM) including tumor cells microscopically infiltrating adjacent brain parenchyma with confirming clean surgical margin by intraoperative margin biopsy is not known. This study was carried out to clarify the therapeutic impact of such resections.

Material and Methods; From June 2002 to December 2014, 90 patients (66 males and 24 females; mean age: 56.7 years) underwent surgical resection for BM. The authors undertook microscopic complete resection, including microscopic infiltrative tumor cells adjacent brain parenchyma, with confirming a pathologically clean surgical margin during surgery for the BMs located in a non-eloquent area in 47 patients (Group A), but in 43 patients, the authors undertook gross complete resection without removal of neighboring brain parenchyma due to their eloquent location (Group B). The two groups were then compared in terms of survival, and local and distant recurrence.

Results; Mean follow-up duration was 18.6 month and 71 patients (78.9%) died during follow-up. Median survival times were 13.1 months in group A and 12.1 months in group B ($p = 0.309$). One-year and 2-year local recurrence rates were 21.2% and 25.8% in group A, and 65.2% and 65.2% in group B, respectively ($p = 0.000$). One-year and 2-year distant recurrence rates were 46.3% and 57.2% in group A, and 33.2% and 33.2% in group B, respectively ($p = 0.140$).

Conclusion; These results suggest that the wide surgical resection of BM including tumor cells infiltrating adjacent brain parenchyma with confirming clean surgical margin renders better local control.

Chapter 3 - This chapter encapsulates the trends of the computer-aided diagnosis (CAD) development for the estimation of tumor malignancy. Due to the high occurrence rate of cancer, more and more abnormal cell growth can appear at any organs in human body. To avoid unnecessary biopsy, the malignancy evaluation should be modeled and acquired via noninvasive examinations. CADs based on medical images are the effective tool for this purpose. Upon the developments of imaging modalities, more and more tumor characteristics can be observed and quantified. As an adjunct to mammography in breast cancer. Ultrasound techniques including B-mode, Doppler, elastogaphy are proposed to extract the physical, mechanical properties, and vessel distribution around tumors. Based on the artificial intelligence classifier, the complementary power of various features can be combined to deal with the heterogeneity of cancer types. These quantitative features can be classified into two categories: morphology and texture features. For ultrasound images, the echogenicities of different tissues are presented by gray-scale pixel values. The gray-scale intensities of region of interest can be analyzed without image segmentation or manual delineation and thus especially convenient for texture analysis. However, different settings or manufactures of ultrasound scanners usually result in different gray-scale distributions for the same tissue. The newly developed intensity-invariant texture features based on multi-resolution and orientations which successfully classified breast tumors into benign and malignant groups with accuracy higher than 80% are introduced as a solution. Finally, the use of CAD can be extended to precision medicine. Gene expression of everyone is quite different due to the inherent and environmental effects. In the past, the researches about gene are isolated to clinical examinations because the cost and the invasive procedures. With the development of image features extracted from medical images such as computed tomography, magnetic resonance imaging, ultrasound, and so on, the correlations between hundreds of quantitative image features and gene expressions are explored. The success of the researches can discover more tumor characteristics from image properties to gene expression for cancer stage estimation, survival rate, and many related issues. The role of CAD would be more important than before because of the computation of more data and more sophisticated techniques.

Chapter 4 - Dendritic cell (DC)-based tumor vaccines called DC therapy are being explored as a promising therapeutic option to stimulate immune responses that recognize and selectively eliminate malignant cells. For successful DC therapy, it is crucial to marshal and orchestrate a vast array of effector cells. These cells include *adaptive immune cells* such as tumor-antigen-specific CD8+ T cells and CD4+ helper T cells, *innate immune cells* such as γδT cells and NK cells, and *innate/adaptive immune cells,* invariant

NKT cells (iNKT) in which DCs play a pivotal role in bridging innate and adaptive immunities. In this study, the authors demonstrate in patients with glioblastoma multiforme (GBM) that copulsing cytomegalovirus derived peptide, pp65 (CMVpp65-peptide)-pulsed IFN-DCs with zoledronate (Z) and α-galactosylceramide (α-GalCer; G) efficiently induces CMVpp65-specific cytotoxic CD8+ T cells through Vγ9γδT cell and iNKT cell expansion. The IFN-DCs derived from patients with GBM used in this study express higher levels of CD56, CD14, and CD36 and lower levels of PDL1 and PDL2 than the most commonly used mature IL-4DCs. The expression of the lymph-node-homing receptor CCR7 on IFN-DCs was up-regulated following their culture with the peptide, Z, and G. In the supernatant of co-culture of lymphocytes and autologous IFN-DCs in the presence of the peptide, Z, and G, higher amounts of Th1 cytokines such as IFNγ and TNFα which are favorable for induction of cytotoxic T cell , higher amounts of IL-18, which up-regulate DC function, and lower amounts of IL-6, which down-regulate DC function, were detected than in the supernatant of co-culture of lymphocytes with autologous IFN-DCs in the presence of the peptide alone. Multifunctional T cells including HLA-A*0201-specific CMVpp65-specific CD8+T cells, Vγ9γδT cells, and iNKT cells efficiently kill HLA-A*0201-positive GBM tumor cell line.

Chapter 5 - The skin is the largest organ in the human body weighing ~3.6 kg and covering ~2m^2 in the average adult. It is the first line of defence against external aggressions and acts as a passive barrier against physical traumas and environmental insults. The fact that healthy skin contains more than twice the number of CD8$^+$ T cells found in the blood (approx. 2x10^{10} cells), underlines the key role of the skin in protection from infection and carcinogens and emphasizes the importance of this population in the maintenance of skin homeostasis. The crucial anti-tumour role played by T cells in the skin is clearly demonstrated by the high rate of skin tumour formation in organ transplant patients who receive T cell suppressive drugs to maintain the integrity of their transplanted organs. These patients show a 10-100 fold increased risk of cutaneous squamous cell carcinoma (SCC) development compared to healthy patients, and indeed, some renal transplant patients currently presenting to the Princess Alexandra Hospital, Brisbane, Australia, require the removal of ~120 primary skin tumours each year. However, although this relationship has been well-documented, it is still very unclear which T cell populations or mechanisms mediate cancer protection in the skin. This chapter will address CD8$^+$ T cell activation and regulation in the skin, paying special attention to what it is known about $CD8^+$ T cell activity and its link with SCC development.

Chapter 6 - Triterpenoids, often referred as terpenes, are compounds of natural and semi-synthetic origin containing a dual five carbon backbone. Triterpenoids have been documented as analgesic, anti-inflammatory, anti-viral, anti-microbial, hepatoprotective, sedative, and cardioprotective in a number of studies. In addition, triterpenoids have been extensively studied as potent anti-cancer agents. Anti-cancer mechanisms of triterpenoid action include blockade of nuclear factor (NF)-κB activation, induction of apoptosis, and suppression of angiogenesis causing mitochondrial dysfunction. Moreover, triterpenoids have been studied, pre clinically, as reversal agents of ABC transporter-mediated multi drug resistance (MDR) in cancer. They have been shown to block the efflux function of a multitude of drug efflux transporters, thereby causing an increase in drug accumulation and cell death. This chapter discusses the authors' current knowledge of the molecular basis of anti-cancer drug resistance and the mechanisms through which triterpenoids modulate ABC transporter-mediated MDR.

Chapter 7 - Heparan sulfate proteoglycans (HSPGs) are glycoproteins, with the common characteristic of containing covalently attached heparan sulfate glycosaminoglycan chains (GAGs). GAGs have specific structural patterns generated through a series of interdependent enzymatic reactions that can involve various isoenzymes with differences in their specificities, responsible for the modification of the structure in physiological and pathological processes. In this light, HSPGS are highly modified in cancer, contributing to tumorigenesis. In fact, the expression of HSPGs is markedly altered during malignant transformation and tumor progression, affecting both the PG core proteins and the GAG chains. Numerous tumours show quantitative and structural alterations of heparan sulphate chains, largely caused by changes in the expression of the enzymes responsible for their biosynthesis, particularly at the fine structure level.

The authors discuss here some of the main regulatory points in HSPG formation and modification, all of which are implicated in cancer development and progression. Numerous tumours show quantitative and structural alterations largely caused by changes in the expression of the enzymes responsible for HSPGs biosynthesis, particularly at the fine structure level. The result is the alteration of the ligand binding sites responsible for directing specific cell signaling effects.

Chapter 8 - Cancer is a multifactorial disease involving network of genes, controlling the functions of the cell. Use of sophisticated tool and techniques in molecular biology revealed the mechanistic binding of numerous genes indulged in the progression of cancer. A wide range of synthetic products was synthesized; whose efficiency decreased the mortality rate from last few decades. Natural products serve as templates to synthesize new efficient products in the cancer treatment. A broad spectrum of antibiotics and drugs were obtained from natural products without any detrimental effect. Among natural products, terpenes emerged as a better class in modulating various signaling pathway in cancer. In cancer, topoisomerases play a crucial role in controlling replication, transcription, and translation process. Topoisomerases regulates the overwinding or underwinding of DNA which regulates the functioning of cell cycle. One of the renowned medicinal mushrooms, *Ganoderma lucidum* targets various pathways in cancer, one among them is apoptosis. Ganoderic acid, triterpenes isolated from *Ganoderma lucidum*, played crucial role in apoptosis pathway were studied in this chapter.

Chapter 9 - The model for cAMP-dependent synaptic plasticity relates the characterization of a noradrenaline-stimulated adenylyl cyclase with DNA unzipping. Specific proteins condition cAMP insertion in specific sites of the DNA structure to direct cellular and synaptic differentiation in brain tissues, also providing coding. Metabolic-dependent ATP binding of Mg^{2+}, could control feedback by inactivating AC dependent formation of cAMP. The level of cAMP and cGMP, which could be assayed in red cells and cerebrospinal fluid, allows a clinical lab diagnostic improvement. Also, provides a relationship of best fitting to cAMP control by binding to DNA. The cAMP level allows the prediction of an inverse relationship between neurodegeneration and cancer. The latter, could be characterized by uncontrolled proliferation, whereas metabolic dominance by stress over a long period of time, may deplete cerebral cAMP.

Chapter 10 - Male breast cancer (MBC) comprises less than 1% of all cancers in men and less than 1% of all breast cancer in United States. In contrast to female breast cancer (FBC), male patients are generally older and have more advanced disease. MBC is rarely detected before age 30 and the mean age is 67 years. The advanced stage at presentation of MBC is thought to be related to thin breast parenchymal tissue in men. The tumors are often low or intermediate grade, with a higher percentage of ER-positive tumors. Patients with MBC routinely receive tamoxifen. All-cause mortality (ACM) is higher than FBC: for example in node-positive patients, all-cause mortality rate at 10-year was 67% in MBC versus 52% in FBC. There is a higher rate of distant recurrence for MBC. Factors such as advanced age, stage, visceral metastasis, triple-negative disease, androgen receptor, high grade, never married, smoking and low income at baseline are known to adversely affect outcome. The survival rates for MBC have lagged behind those for FBC. Prognosis may improve with more research on MBC in the future.

In: Horizons in Cancer Research. Volume 63 ISBN: 978-1-53610-013-6
Editor: Hiroto S. Watanabe

Chapter 1

NEW PARADIGMS IN THE MANAGEMENT OF BRAIN METASTASES FROM NON-SMALL CELL LUNG CANCER (NSCLC)

***Ng Chai Ching*[1], *Chen Fangxia*[2] *and Alex Chang*[3]**
[1]National Healthcare group, Tan Tock Seng Hospital, Singapore
[2]Johns Hopkins Singapore
[3]Sydney Kimmel Comprehensive, Cancer Centre
Johns Hopkins University

ABSTRACT

Brain metastases (BMs) from NSCLC cause significant morbidity and mortality for patients and major challenge in the management and care. BMs with increasing incidence in the current era of targeted therapy and immunotherapy has become a more important clinical issue. This is because patients tend to live longer from more effective therapy. MRI or CT of the brain has been incorporated in the routine tests of staging newly diagnosed NSCLC. Thus more asymptomatic BMs have been discovered. Therefore BMs have attracted a lot of attention from academic and private oncologists and the management has transformed to new paradigms. Whole brain radiation (WBRT) is no longer the standard therapy for BMs. Once the BMs are confirmed, treatment is often based on the presence of driver mutations of primary NSCLC mass and if the mutation is drugable or not. Tyrosine kinase inhibitor is usually used to treat NSCLC with a sensitive mutation. Stereotactic Radiation (SRS) has gradually replaced WBRT especially in patients with less than 10 metastatic lesions. Radiation as the first line therapy is often reserved for NSCLC patients without driver mutations. This chapter reviews the most recent advances in the management, analyses the best possible treatment in each scenario, and discusses the future research direction on BMs from NSCLC.

Keywords: brain metastases (BMs), non-small cell lung cancer (NSCLC), tyrosine kinase inhibitor (TKI), diver mutations, whole brain radiotherapy (WBRT), stereotactic radiation (SRS)

INTRODUCTION

Lung cancer remains the leading cause of cancer-related death worldwide. It affected about 224,000 people in United States in 2014, with 5-year survivorship of 16.8% [1]. Its high mortality is partly related to the presence of metastases at diagnosis, the increased incidence of relapse following treatment, and resistance to standard therapies.

Lung cancer can further classified into small cell lung cancer (SCLC) and non-small cell lung cancer (NSCLC), which consists of squamous cell lung cancer (SCC), lung adenocarcinomas (LAC) and large-cell carcinomas.

The incidence of BMs in NSCLC has increased due to improved imaging and better systemic control. Currently, about 10% of NSCLC patients will have BMs on diagnosis while up to 40% develop BMs during the course of their disease [2]. Such patients suffer from considerable morbidity and mortality even with good systemic disease control due to loss of independence from cognitive and physical impairment. Traditionally, BM has been a poor prognostic factor portending a median life expectancy of 4 months even after WBRT [3].

Recently, advances in molecular biology of NSCLC have led to interest in the use of molecularly target agents in the treatment of brain metastases in these patients. Biomarkers such as mutations in EGFR, KRAS, TP53, ALK and BRCA1 have been identified to have prognostic and therapeutic value

[4, 5]. Tyrosine kinase inhibitors (TKIs) against specific driver mutations have been developed and become the first treatment choice for patients with metastatic NSCLC. Response rates of 75-89% in EGFR-mutated NSCLC patients with BMs treated with EGFR-TKIs have been reported [6]. Thus if a treatable molecular alteration like ALK translocation or EGFR mutation is

diagnosed, treatment with a targeted agent like ALK-TKI or EGFR-TKI would represent the most efficacious treatment. Hence brain irradiation is usually delayed until clinical/radiological progression occurs, which could prevent/delay the exposure to the side effects of irradiation. However, poor penetration of TKI to the brain due to blood-brain barrier (BBB) remains an issue in the treatment of BMs. For example, poor BBB penetration has been postulated to be the cause of CNS progression of ALK positive patients on crizotinib [5, 7]. Second generation ALK inhibitors agents (e.g., ceritinib, alectinib) may be potentially more viable treatment options in these patients, although larger phase III trials are required to determine their efficacy [7]. In the meantime, radiation therapy to brain has also changed due to the availability of SRS as being more precise, efficient and less toxic. So SRS has been advocated as the first choice of radiation for selected patients without actionable driver mutations. Here we try to present the up-to-date study results.

PATIENTS WITH DRUGABLE DRIVER MUTATION

No Prior TKI Therapy

Epidermal growth factor receptor (EGFR)

10-50% patients with NSCLCs have somatic mutations in the epidermal growth factor receptor (EGFR) tyrosine kinase domain [8], more frequently observed in non-smokers, adenocarcinomas and women, and occur in 50% of Asians and only 10% of non-Asians. These mutations mainly occur as deletions in exon 19 or as a single missense mutation at position 858 on exon 21. Patients with these mutations generally responded well to EGFR-TKIs, e.g., Erlotinib (Tarceva) and Gefitinib (Iressa) [9-11].

1st Generation EGFR-TKI: Gefitinib, Erlotinib

Gefitinib

Gefitinib (Iressa) was the 1st oral EGFR inhibitor that come on the market. According to Iressa® Survival Evaluation in Lung Cancer (ISEL) study (Trial 709) gefitinib didn't significantly prolong survival in overall study population or in patients with adenocarcinoma [12], except in 2 specific patient subsets: patients of Asian origin (median, 9.5 versus 5.5 months, respectively; HR, 0.66; p = .010) and never-smokers (median, 8.9 versus 6.1 months, respectively; HR, 0.67; p = .012). Gefitinib may not have free access the brain barrier as imatinib, the small low-molecular weight TKI that is shown to have limited brain penetration [13]. Its level in the CSF is about 1% of plasma levels and is reported to be insufficient for tumour inhibition [14]. There are several reports that gefitinib is effective in BMs for several tumours however this may be partly contributed by sensitivity of cancer cells to the drug and BBB disruption caused by tumour invasion [15].

Erlotinib

Erlotinib level in the CSF is about 5% of plasma levels and has been reported to be sufficient to inhibit the EGFR receptor. In a review article by Cohen et al., [16] erlotinib demonstrated a survival advantage when compared to placebo in patients who failed at least one prior chemotherapy regime; 6.67 months versus 4.70 months, respectively. It was also superior to placebo for progression-free survival (PFS) and objective response rate. And in contrary to ISEL results, it appeared to prolong survival for most of the other patient subsets, although a larger study is needed to draw a definite conclusion. The difference in efficacy between gefitinib and erlotinib may be partly contributed by the fact that erlotinib was dosed at its maximum-tolerated dose (MTD) [8], while gefitinib was dosed at about one third of its MTD [17].

2nd Generation EGFR-TKI: Afatinib

The targeted agents afatinib and gefitinib block key pathways involved in tumour growth and spread. They have both been approved for the treatment of naive patients, based on the results of Phase III trials, confirming their superiority compared to chemotherapy.

In two large phase III studies (LUX-Lung 3 and LUX-Lung 6), afatinib was used as first-line treatment for EGFR mutant NSCLC and was shown to have significant improvement in PFS rates, objective response rates and patient-reported outcomes compared with platinum-based chemotherapy. In the subgroup analyses of these two studies which included EGFR-mutant NSCLC patients with BMs, afatinib had significantly improved PFS and objective response rates with objective response rate of 72.9% (35 of 48 patients) [18].

Anaplastic lymphoma kinase (ALK)

3-4% of patients with NSCLC have chromosomal rearrangements of ALK. ALK-positive patients are highly responsive to ALK-TKI. ALK-TKIs have been shown to have more superior PFS to chemotherapy as the first line treatment in patients with positive ALK rearrangement NSCLC

1st Generation ALK Inhibitors (ALK-i) Crizotinib

Crizotinib is a small molecule TKI with activity against the receptor tyrosine kinases ALK, ROS1 and MET [19-21]. It showed superiority to cytotoxic chemotherapy in advanced ALK-positive NSCLC with 65-74% of patients achieving a response [22, 23]. However most patients tend to relapse within 1st year of treatment and the most common site of relapse is CNS. This probably reflects poor penetration of crizotinib through the BBB and failure to achieve therapeutic drug concentrations in the CNS [24]. There are a few reports which suggested poor CSF penetration ability of crizotinib in view of its poor CSF-to-plasma ratio [24]. However significant CNS radiographic responses to crizotinib have been described, which may be contributed by factors other than pharmacokinetic resistance alone. In the PROFILE 1005 and 1007 trials, the intracranial response rate was 18% in untreated BMs and 33% in previously treated BMs by radiation [25]. Clinical benefit of continuing crizotinib after disease progression was also noted [26, 27].

2nd Generation ALK-i

2nd generation ALK-i may have further improvement against ALK positive NSCLC [28, 29].

Ceritinib

Ceritinib demonstrated about 20-fold greater efficacy than crizotinib and prolonged activity in xenograft models [30, 31]. In ASCEND-1 trial, it showed about 54.5% of intracranial response rate in patients receiving oral ceretinib at a recommended dose of 750mg/day in the dose-escalation and expansion phases.[32].

Alectinib

It was shown that alectinib crosses BBB efficiently with about 75% of patients with measurable CNS disease at baseline achieved an intracranial response while 25% of patients with measurable and non-measurable CNS lesions achieved a complete response [33, 34]. In a study of 52 patients with measurable or non-measurable CNS metastases at baseline, intracranial responses were achieved in 67% patients with previously untreated CNS lesions [35]. Its superiority compared to crizotinib was further supported by its ability to salvage CNS relapses, including leptomeningeal disease (LM), after failure of crizotinib and ceritinib [35]. Alectinib is well tolerated, with most adverse events being grade 1 or 2 (mostly nausea and diarrhea), and less patients required dose deduction, interruption and withdrawal. Only about 6% of patients had a rise in aminotransferase levels to grade 3 or 4, which required interruption of treatment.

With Prior Therapy

EGFR

EGFR positive NSCLC patients can acquire EGFR-TKI resistance as they develop secondary mutations during therapy, [36] e.g., T790M substitution in EGFR exon 20 and MET amplification.

About 1/3 of patients developed CNS metastases after initial EGFR-TKIs treatment [37-39].

1st Generation: Erlotinib/Gefitinib

Erlotinib

Clarke et al., reported that daily dosing of erlotinib 150mg was inadequate to achieve sufficient CSF concentration to kill EGFR mutant NSCLC cells [40]. But these CNS metastases may retain EGFR-TKI sensitivity if sufficient drug concentrations can be achieved in brain parenchyma as CNS metastases do not consistently harbour acquired resistance mutations found in synchronous disease outside the CNS. [40, 41] Christian et al., [42] recruited patients with worsening CNS metastases during or following treatment with standard dosing of EGFR-TKI. They gave these patients erlotinib at approximately 1500mg once dose per week. They found the high dose pulsing erlotinib was safe with a 67% response in CNS disease. Based on RECIST evaluation, even when systemic resistance had developed and confirmed, the median overall survival was 12 months.

Gefitinib

In a previous case report studying the response and resistance of NSCLC patient with EGFR mutation and BM, gefitinib as a single agent was increased from 500mg up to 1250mg per day over the course of 2 months. With the increment in gefitinib dosage, the CSF concentrations of gefitinib were over 40nM, exceeding that of in vitro IC50 in H3255 and DFCILU-011, 2 NSCLC cell lines with sensitizing mutations in the EGFR [35, 43]. These patients' CNS symptoms had improved and CSF cytology no longer showed evidence of lung cancer cells. Post-mortem studies of the patients showed development of T790M resistance mutation in the systemic sites but not in the CNS metastases [41]. In the absence of other effective treatment options, it's reasonable to consider the use of high dose gefitinib at 750mg daily for 14 days followed by 500mg for 14 days. Prior post mortem examinations revealed that CNS metastases of these patients will often remain sensitive to EGFR-TKI therapy [41, 44]. This study has demonstrated a consistent ability of high dose gefitinib to achieve an adequate gefitinib CSF concentration to treat LM [45]. In a phase I trial of high dose gefitinib for NSCLC patients with in LMs (with or without prior response to EGFR-TKI) conducted by Jackman et. Al [41], diarrhea was the most common drug-related toxicity in patients receiving gefitinib 750mg, with one case of grade 3 toxicity. Other toxicities noted with this dose including rash, fatigue, nausea, vomiting, elevated alkaline phosphatase (either grade 1 or 2). For the gefitinib 1000mg cohort [46], there was one drug-limiting toxicity (DLTs) after completing 1 cycle of therapy: a patient with Sjogren's syndrome was found to have disease progression in CNS and systematically and died of systemic lung cancer progression 3 weeks later. The maximum tolerated dose for the gefitinib schedule was not formally defined, with the 750mg dose level was well tolerated without DLT, as the trial was subsequently closed due to slow accrual.

2nd Generation: Afatinib

NSCLC patients who continued to progress with CNS metastases despite at least one line of chemotherapy and one line of EGFR-TKI treatment seem to respond well to afatinib. The rate of both systemic and CNS disease control were high [47]. Afatinib remains potent at relatively low concentration, but very little is known about the ability of afatinib to penetrate CNS. The plasma and CSF concentrations of afatinib was measured in one patient in compassionate use program (CUP) and gave a CSF to plasma ratio of <1%. By correlating the clinical improvement and disappearance of tumour cells in CSF , it suggested that the dose reached was sufficient to inhibit tumour growth. The possible speculations including lower CSF protein concentrations than that of blood, so ratios of free concentrations would be higher; afatinib has a high affinity to EGFR which would be overexpressed in the tumour tissues; and there are possible distribution processes in the CNS which could lead to higher concentrations at the target tissue [47]. On the other hand, afatinib has a lower in vitro inhibitory concentration compared to that of gefitinib and erlotinib [48, 49]. Thus it may remain effective in the CSF after resistance to other TKIs has developed, and can be potentially used to treat CNS metastases despite incomplete penetration of the BBB. This is supported by regression of CNS metastases observed during afatinib CUP. The overall cerebral response rate to afatinib treatment was 35% [47].

3rd Generation: Osimertinib

There are ongoing trials on the new 3rd generation EGFR TKI, osimertinib (AstraZenaca). In a combined analysis of patients from AURA and AURA 2 trials, 39% patients had CNS metastases and the ORR of those patients was 56%, compared to 64% of those without CNS metastases [50].

2nd Generation ALK-i: Ceritinib/Alectinib

Ceritinib

Ceritinib has demonstrated an ORR of 50% in patients who were previously treated with ALK inhibitors compared to 69.2% of BMs patients who had not received prior ALK inhibitor [51]. Its use for ALK positive NSCLC patients who have progressed or were intolerant to crizotinib was approved in April 2014 in view of similar median PFS compared to crizotinib-naïve patients [29].

Alectinib

Alectinib has demonstrated efficacy in salvaging CNS disease in patients treated with both crizotinib and ceretinib [52]. An intracranial response rate of 52% was observed when alectinib was given to crizotinib resistant or intolerant NSCLC patients with BMs [53].

Overall

More studies are needed to establish whether the molecular determinants of ALK-I resistance are the same in CNS and extracranial disease and also the optimal sequence of ALK-I [47].

Table 1. Overall response rate for various classes of TKI in NSCLC with BMs

	Without prior TKI therapy	With prior TKI therapy
EGFR TKI		
1st generantion		
Gefitinib	60-80%	-
Erlotinib	60-80%	67%
2nd generation		
Afatinib	72.9%	35%
3rd generation		
Osimertinib	-	56%
ALK TKI		
1st generantion		
Crizotinib	**18%**	**-**
2nd generation		
Ceritinib	**54.5%**	**50%**
Alectinib	**67%**	**52%**

Genomic Precision Medicine

Although the genomics-based-therapeutic selection has shown to have improved response rates over conventional therapy [54, 55], only a small portion of patients harbour these molecular alterations, which is drugable. A more thorough understanding of molecular landscapes of tumour types offer opportunities to discover driver events and also to predict therapeutic strategies based on individual tumour biology. Example, the discovery of previously 'undruggable' genes such as Kirsten rat sarcoma viral oncogene homolog (KRAS), serine/threonine kinase 11 (STK11/LKB1) and tumour protein p53 (TP53).

Lung Adenocarcinoma (LAC)

LAC is the most common histological subtype of lung cancer which are highly heterogenous with high rates of somatic mutations and genomic rearrangements [56]. Genomic mutations such as EGFR and ALK are prominent in LAC. Identification of the genomic mutations and pathways alteration is likely to help in determining which therapy is more likely to elicit a response.

Squamous Cell lung Carcinoma (SCC)

SCC is the 2nd most common type of NSCLC behind LAC. Targeted therapy for EGFR and ALK is hardly effective in squamous cell lung cancer as these genomic mutations are not common in SCC [54, 55].

Other Emerging Targets in LAC

- Ret Proto-oncogene (RET)

Besides EGFR and ALK, RET is another genetic rearrangement found in patients with LAC. It is responsible for encoding a receptor tyrosine kinase involved in neural crest development, growth and differentiation [57]. Besides NSCLC, it is also implicated in diseases like medullary thyroid carcinoma, multiple endocrine neoplasia (MEN type IIA and IIB) and Hirschsprung disease [57]. There are limited options available for patients positive for RET rearrangement. Carbozantinib (XL-184), a multi-TKI and RET inhibitor, is currently undergoing phase II clinical trials to determine its efficacy in RET fusion-positive advanced NSCLC [58]. Vandetanib which is a RET/VEGF/EGFR inhibitor is approved for treatment of medullary thyroid carcinoma. There are ongoing studies for small-molecule inhibitors like Ponatinib, Levatinibb, MGCD516 and Sunitinib.

- Kirsten Rat Sarcoma Viral Oncogene Homolog (KRAS)

KRAS functions as a molecular switch that propagates signal transduction pathways and is associated with tumour-related signalling pathways including MAPK signalling, RAC, RAL signalling etc. [59]. It is prevalent not only in LAC but also in other malignancies such as pancreatic cancer (about 95% of cases) [58].

- Tumour Protein p53 (TP53)

TP53 mutation or deletion, according to TCGA, is found in 90% of SCC and 46% of LAC [60, 61].

There are limited therapeutic options for patients with TP53 mutation. To date, therapeutic strategies that were being explored including reintroduction of the wild type gene for TP53 deletion and small molecules that inhibit the growth of cancer harbouring TP53 mutations etc.

- Serine/Threonine Kinase II (STK II)/Liver Kinase B1 (LKB1)

STKII/LKB1 mutations are found in both familial and sporadic pattern. More recent TCGA analyses showed that LKBI mutations are primarily a characteristic of LAC [56. 60, 61] and is found between 15-30% of LAC tumours.

- Other Molecular Targets in LAC

About 10% of LAC patients harboured BRAF mutations. BRAF inhibitors, Vemurafenib was shown to be effective in LAC cases with BRAF mutations [62]. Meanwhile, hepatocyte growth factor receptor (HGFR/MET) occur in 12% LAC cases [60].

Other Emerging Targets in SCC

- Fibroblast Growth Factor 1 (FGFR1)

FGFR1-4 are a member of tyrosine kinases family that are involved in development, angiogenesis and proliferation of cells [63]. FGFR1 is the one most commonly dysregulated in SCC by receptor activation or amplification and its presence is associated with poor prognosis [63-66]. AZD4547 is TKI specific to FGFR 1-4 which showed cytotoxic and cytostatic effects in cell lines with FGFR amplifications [67]. It also demonstrated mild inhibition of VEGF4 [67].

- Phosphatidylinositol-4,5-bisphosphate 3-kinase, catalytic subunit alpha (PIK3CA)

The receptor tyrosine kinases activate the P13K which will in turn activates the AKT/MTOR pathway to drive cell growth and survival. Mutational inactivation of tumour suppressor PTEN, the main antagonistic regulators of P13K will lead to hyperactivation of P13K signalling and increased cell growth [68].

- TP53 Mutation is found in about 90% of SCC and its high prevalence may dictate the use of TP53 therapeutics, as discussed above.
- Other genomic alterations such as EGFR, ERRB2, KRAS, BRAF and MET account for 3-9% of SCC and could be treated with targeted therapeutic strategies as discussed previously [60].

RADIOTHERAPY

For the last several decades, WBRT and surgery have been the main treatment options for BMs from NSCLC. However, the development of methods of treatment using radiosurgery devices “Gamma Knife”, “Cyber Knife” has significantly changed the results of treatment of patients with BMs, which allowed formulating new principles of treatment of this group of patients.

Whole-Brain Radiotherapy (WBRT)

Sine 1980s, WBRT has been the cornerstone in the treatment for multiple BMs from variable primary tumors including lung cancer [69-71]. Indications [72] for WBRT include multiple BMs (4 or more metastases), oligometastases (1-3 metastases) with poorly controlled systemic disease, oligometastases too large (>4cm) for SRS, re-irradiation after late WBRT failure, and after surgery or SRS.

Historically, radiotherapy directed to the whole brain developed for several practical reasons. Without high quality radiological scans, physicians in early days were unable to accurately localize or selectively target individual lesion. However, a clinical rationale for WBRT emerged gradually: in addition to palliating macroscopic metastatic lesions, WBRT could also sterilize microscopic metastases invisible in the scans and reduce risk of further significant recurrence.

Retrospective studies have suggested benefit of WBRT of improving median survival, from 1-2 month without WBRT to 3-6 month with it [73]. However, patients with BMs should be treated with individual approaches taking into account prognostic factors that influence survival. Whether or not to treat with WBRT vs best supportive care (BSC) for patients with BMs from NSCLC has been addressed in the recent phase III randomized trial (QUARTZ trial) [74]. Interim data from the trial showed there was no difference in overall survival (49 days vs 51 days) between WBRT arm and BSC arm. Interestingly, these data was based on 151 patient with half of these patients were RTOG RPA class 3 (KPS <70) and approximately 25% of patients in WBRT arm did not receive radiation or received less than the intended fractions. These data suggested that BSC is a reasonable choice in patients with baseline poor prognosis. Further efforts are required to improve identifications of patients who are likely to benefit from WBRT, e.g by refining survival prediction tools.

A number of studies have attempted to identify the optimal dose and fractionation of WBRT in the setting of BMs. Cumulative experiences showed that 30Gy in 10 daily fractions is the most widely accepted, tolerable and effective fractionation. A Cochrane review [75] in 2012 found that there was no significant benefit of altered dose fractionation schedules as compare to the conventional scheme (30Gy in 10 daily fractions) for overall survival. There was also no improvement in symptom control nor neurologic improvement among the different dose-fractionation schemes as compared to the standard 30Gy in 10 daily fractions. In the other hand, study [76] showed that daily fractions of more than 3Gy may cause acute radiation toxicity with neurologic deterioration in patients with extensive pretreatment edema.

Role of adding radiosensitizers , such as motexafin gadolinium [77-79] or efaproxrial [80, 81], has been studied in several randomized phase III trials, but none has shown to confer additional benefit to WBRT in either overall survival times or brain tumor response rates. Others including lonidamine [82], metronidazole [83], misonidazole [84], bromodeoxyuridine85 have also been studied. All showed similar negative results.

The most concerning toxicity associated with WBRT is irreversible neurocognitive dysfunction in long-term survivors. However, in patients with BMs from stage IV NSCLC, overall prognosis is poor and tumor progression affects neurocognitive function adversely more frequently than radiotherapy-induced neurotoxicity.

Nevertheless, neurocognitive dysfunction following WBRT is widely accepted as real and clinically relevant. Several strategies have evolved to prevent WBRT related neurocognitive dysfunction.

Hippocampus-avoidance WBRT (HA-WBRT) is a novel radiation technique devised to spare critical hippocampal area and has shown to have potential to reduce WBRT-related memory loss [86, 87]. The rationale behind HA-WBRT is that the formation of new memory has been associated with a lifelong mitotically active and radiosensitive compartment of neural stem cell located in the hippocampal dentate gyrus and injury to this neural stem-cell compartment has been hypothesized to be central to the pathogenesis of radiation-induced early cognitive decline. A single arm phase II study (RTOG 0933) [87] confirmed HA-WBRT technique was associated with preservation of memory and quality of life as compared to historical control of patients treated with WBRT without hippocampal avoidance, with a mean relative decline in delayed recall is 7% in HA-WBRT treated patients, vs 30% in historical controls. Phase III studies are still ongoing.

Another strategy to reduce radiation-related neurocognitive dysfunction is the addition of neuroprotective agent during WBRT. Several agents have been tried, such as donepezil [88] and mamantine [89], but none showed to have convincing success.

With the rapid development in targeted therapy, WBRT has also been used in combination with systemic therapy, e.g., with TKIs in EGFR mutant NSCLC with BM. In preclinical models, overexpression of EGFR is associated with radiation resistance, while EFGR signaling blockage sensitizes EGFR-mutant cells to radiation [90, 91]. Hence, it has been hypothesized that concurrent EGFR inhibition and WBRT may synergistic and potentially improve survival. Retrospective studies and small prospective studies [92-94] showed that WBRT with concomitant targeted therapy TKIs could effectively and safely control intracranial lesions in NSCLC with BM patients, as well as improve overall survival of these patients. In a meta-analysis, Zheng et al., [95] included 7 trials involving total of 622 patients to efficacy and safety of combining WBRT with gefitinib/erlotinib for treatment of BM from NSCLC. They found that compared with WBRT alone or WBRT plus chemotherapy, WBRT plus gefitinib/erotinib could significantly improve response rate (Odds ratio,OR = 2.16, 95% CI: 1.35-3.47, p = 0.001) and overall survival (HR 0.72, 95% CI: 0.58-0.89; p = 0.002). And except for rash (OR = 7.96, 95% CI: 2.02-31.34; p = 0.003) and myelosuppression (OR = 0.19, 95% CI: 0.07-0.51; p = 0.001), there were no significant differences in adverse events (grade III-IV). However, further large randomized, prospective studies are warranted to confirm the clinical efficacy of RT with concurrent TKI in the treatment of NSCLC with brain metastases.

Stereotactic Radiosurgery (SRS)

SRS was developed as an alternate ablative treatment for surgically inaccessible deep brain lesions. Using devices, such as "Gamma Knife" or "Cyber Knife," SRS precisely delivers high dose of forced radiation to target volume with a rapid dose fall-off, while contributing minimal dose to surrounding tissues. SRS was initially studied as a boost in combination with WBRT, and the addition of SRS to WBRT was hypothesized to improve outcomes.

In 1999, Kondziolka D et al., [96], conducted the first randomized trial evaluating the role of adding SRS boost to WBRT versus WBRT alone, in patients with 2-4 BMs. The study was stopped at an interim evaluation at 60% accrual because of significant benefit of local control of brain lesions noted in WBRT+SRS arm (Table 2), with a median time to local failure was 6 months in WBRT arm vs 36 months in WBRT+SRS arm(p = .0005). Though this was a small trial with only 27 patient enrolled before ending of study, it did show the promising treatment role of SRS in limited BMs.

In the subsequent relative large randomized RTOG 9508 trial [97], total of 331 patients (211 out of 331 had lung cancer) with limited (1-3) BMs were allocated to WBRT alone or WBRT plus SRS group. This study showed that there was a survival advantage in WBRT plus SRS arm for patients with a single BM (4.9 months vs 6.5 months, p = 0.0393), but not for those with 2-3

BMs. However, patients in SRS group were more likely to have a stable or improved Karnofsky Performance Status (KPS) at 6 month's follow-up than patients in WBRT alone group (43% vs 27%, p = 0.03). Hence, the author concluded that WBRT with SRS should be the standard treatment for patients with single unresectable BM and considered for patients with 2 or 3 BMs.

Table 2. Randomized trials evaluating role of SRS

Trials	no. of BM	no. of patients		Median survival (m)			time to local failure (m)			local failure rate at 1 year (%)	
		WBRT alone	WBRT + SRS	WBRT alone	WBRT + SRS	significance (p)	WBRT alone	WBRT + SRS	significance (p)	WBRT alone	WBRT + SRS
Kondziolke D, et al, 1999	2-4	14	13	7.5	11	0.22	6 (95 % CI: 3.5-8.5)	36 (95% CI: 15.6–57)	0,0005	100%	8%
Andrews DW, et al., (RTOG 9508),2004	1-3	164	167	4.9 (for single BM)	6.5(for single BM)	0.0393	-	-	-	-	-

Trials	no. of BM	no. of patients		Median survival (m)			local failure rate at 1 year (%)		
		SRS alone	SRS+ WBRT	SRS alone	SRS+ WBRT	significance (p)	SRS alone	SRS+ WBRT	significance (p)
Aoyama H et al., 2006	1-4	67	65	7.5	8.0	0.42	76.4%	46.8%	<0.01

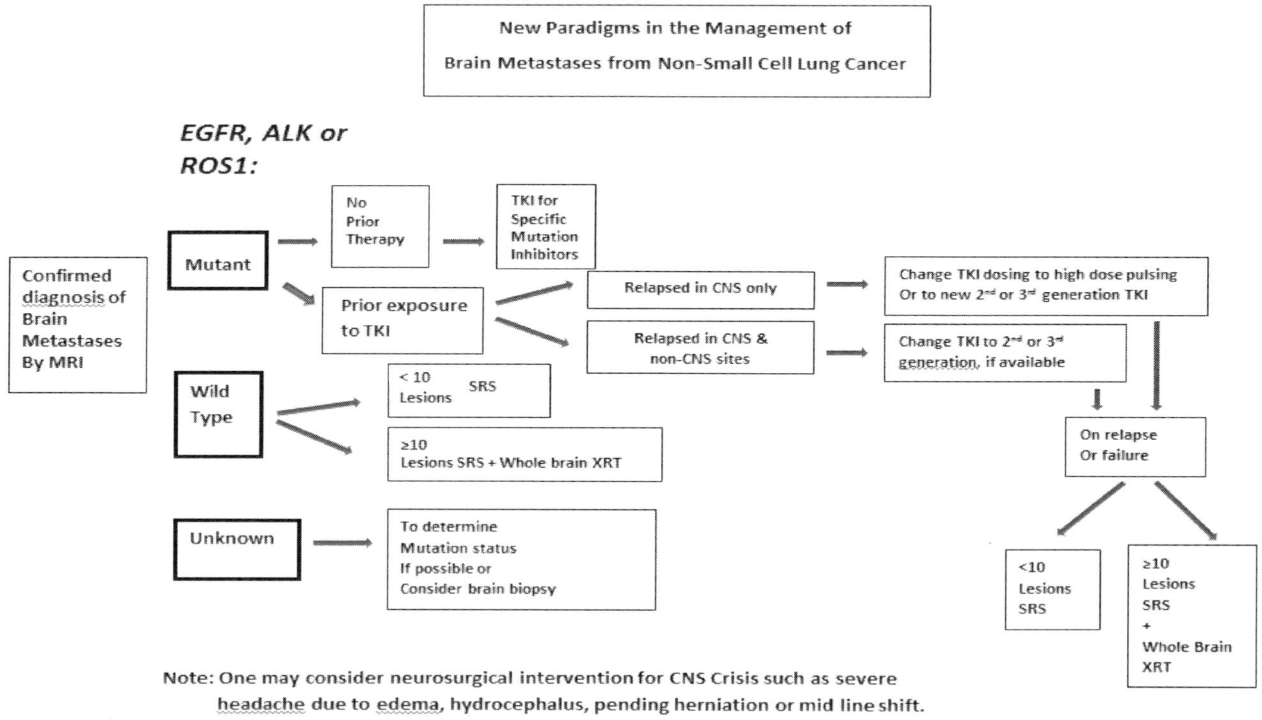

Figure 1. New paradigms in the management of brain metastases from NSCLC.

Note: Though existing randomized trials confirmed role of SRS for patients with up to 4 brain lesions. There is a trend toward using SRS in patients with up to 10 brain lesions.

With the encouraging local control seen with SRS, interest grew in applying SRS in the initial management to avoid or delay WBRT. This was addressed in a randomized controlled trial by Aoyama et al., [98] in 2006, where 132 patients (88 of 132 had NSCLC) with 1-4 BMs were randomly assigned to either WBRT plus SRS or SRS alone. There was no significant survival or functional difference between two groups, but intracranial relapse occurred considerably more frequently in those who did not receive WBRT. Salvage treatment is frequently required when up-front WBRT is not used.

Similar results were found in the phase III EORTC 22952-26001 study [99], where 359 patients with 1-3 BMs WHO PS 0-2 (roughly

KPS >60%), stable disease and who had total surgical resection or SRS as initial local therapy for BMs was randomly allocated to WBRT or observation group. Though adjuvant WBRT reduces intracranial relapses, but fails to improve overall survival. The authors concluded that WBRT could be withheld in good performance status patients with 1-3 BMs initially managed with surgery or SRS, provided close follow-up was performed.

Interestingly, in the secondary analysis of same trial published in Jul 2015 [100], Aoyama et al., utilized diagnosis-specific Graded Prognostic Assessment (DS-GPA) and post-stratifed 88 NSCLC patients into favorable prognosis group (DS-GPA 2.5-4.0) and unfavorable prognosis group(DS-GPA 0.5-2.0). In the secondary analysis, significantly better overall survival was observed in DS-GPA 2.5-4.0 group in WBRT+ SRS vs SRS alone, with a median survival of 16.7 months vs 10.6 months ($P = 0.04$). However, no such difference was observed in the DS-GPA 0.5-2.0 group. This benefit could be explained by differing brain tumor recurrence rates, in that the prevention against recurrence by WBRT had more significant impact in the favorable prognosis group.

In another randomized control trial, Chang et al., [101] compared neurocognition in patients with BMs treated with SRS vs SRS plus WBRT and found that as compared to SRS plus WBRT group was more likely to show learning and memory decline at 4 month.

Based on above data, a strategy of initial treatment with SRS in appropriately selected patients has gained in popularity, with the aim of avoiding or deferring WBRT in an effort to avoid neurocognitive dysfunction. Furthermore, a recent cost-effectiveness study [102] also showed that first-line SRS alone was more cost-effective despite an increased need for salvage therapy. Further evidence also gained from a meta-analysis published in Mar 2015 [103]. In the meta-analysis, Sahgal et al., found that age was a significant effect modifier, favoring SRS alone in patients $\leq$ 50 years of age with a survival advantage, while no significant difference were observed in older patients. In addition, the initial omission of WBRT did not impact distant brain relapse rate.

Although evidence is less clear, upfront SRS with avoidance of WBRT has been used in patients with greater number of brain metastases. Retrospective studies [104] suggest SRS could be an effective strategy in patients with up to 10 brain metastases. More recently, a Japanese multi-institutional prospective observational cohort study [105] showed that SRS alone as initial treatment for patients with 5-10 brain metastases had non inferior survival outcome compared to patients with 2-4 BMs. Further randomized data are required to support role of SRS alone as the initial management in patient with more than 4 BMs.

SURGICAL THERAPY

Patients with a single BM present a special oncologic situation, as they have a better prognosis and may benefit from more intensive local therapy designed to provide more durable local control, leading a rationale for surgical resection of the metastasis. Dated back to 1990s, there were 3 randomized controlled trials [106-108] that assessed the benefit of surgical resection in addition to WBRT for single BM (Patchell et al., 1990; Vecht et al., 1993; Mintz et al., 1996). Two of these studies [106, 107] showed a statistically significant improvement in overall survival for patients managed with surgical resection followed by WBRT compared with WBRT alone. However, the survival advantage was not observed in the third trial reported by Mintz et al., [108]. The lack of benefit may be related to a higher percentage of patients with worse KPS and more extra cranial metastases.

As the value of surgical resection for single BM was widely accepted, subsequent trials were developed to evaluate the additional value of WBRT post-surgical resection. In a multi-center randomized controlled trial, Patchell et al., [109] randomly assigned 95 patients with single BM to surgery alone or surgery followed by WBRT. WBRT reduced intracranial recurrence and neurologic death, but did not improve overall survival. Till now, there is still controversy over the role of "adjuvant" WBRT after surgical resection.

With evolving of SRS and given its less-invasive nature, it has been evaluated as another option for patients with single BM. In RTOG 9508 trial [97] as discussed above, there is survival benefit for patient with single BM treated with SRS plus WBRT compared with WBRT alone. Retrospective studies [110-112] indicated SRS and surgery provide an equivalent benefit in conjunction with WBRT for single BM, though randomized controlled data are still lacking.

Surgery is advantageous for decompression of a symptomatic lesion and for establishing a diagnosis in the absence of more accessible site for biopsy. However, surgery may not be a good option for a lesion in a critical or deep/inaccessbile area such as brainstem metastasis. In addition, it involves hospitalization and recovery time that may delay initiation of systemic therapy, such as chemotherapy or immunotherapy. Radiotherapy is a noninvasive technique and more cost-effective than surgical resection. However, SRS is not suitable for lesions larger than 4cm in maximal diameter or for those with significant mass effect which require urgent decompression.

PRINCIPLES FOR MANAGEMENT OF NON-SMALL CELL LUNG CA WITH BRAIN METASTASES

The core principle in management of NSCLC patients with asymptomatic BMs is to determine on patient's driver mutation status e.g., EGFR/ALK/ROS1 etc. If such driver mutation exists and patient doesn't receive any prior TKI therapy, TKI for specific mutation inhibitor should be the 1st line treatment. However for patients who have had prior TKI exposure, it's reasonable to switch to 2nd or 3rd generation TKI or change the TKI to high dosing pulsing as mentioned previously.

If the driver mutation is not detected, the management will depend largely on the number of brain metastases. Most of the studies support the use of SRS in patients with $\leq$4 brain lesions however there are smaller trials which recommend the use of SRS in patients with <10 brain lesions as well. For those patients with >10 brain lesions, the standard treatment would be SRS with whole brain RT.

In situations where the status of driver mutation is unknown, we would suggest to determine patient's driver mutation status whenever possible or to consider brain biopsy as it has a tremendous impact on patient's subsequent management.

FUTURE RESEARCH DIRECTIONS

Traditional modalities such as surgery, WBRT and SRS still remain the mainstay of treatment for such patients. Patients with oligometastatic disease may benefit from surgical resection or definitive radiation therapy [113], while patients with positive driver mutations BMs may benefit from specific targeted TKIs [114].

New developments in our understanding of the molecular biology of NSCLC may help drive the development of new therapeutic agents through genomic studies. Recent advances in the understanding of cancer immune escape system lead to the development of novel immunotherapy agents that can restore patient's immune response to cancer cells. Immunotherapy with immune checkpoints inhibitors have shown promising results in treatment of NSCLC [115]. Monoclonal antibodies against programmed death-1, Nivolumab and Pembrolizumab, have been shown to have favorable profile in patient with chemotherapy refractory advanced NSCLC in phase 3 studies [116-118]. Compared with second line docetaxel, Nivolumab had superior outcome in overall survival (9.2 months vs. 6.0 months in squamous NSCLC; 12.2 month vs. 9.4 months in nonsquamous NSCLC) and response rate (20% vs 9% in squamous NSCLC, $p = 0.008$; 19% vs 12% in nonsquamous NSCLC, $p = 0.02$) in both squamous and nonsquamous NSCLC [116, 117]. Similarly, Pembrolizumab has been shown to prolong overall survival as compared to docetaxel, 10.4 months with pembrolizumab 2 mg/kg vs, 12.7 months with pembrolizumab 10 mg/kg vs. 8.5 months with docetaxel (HR 0.71, 95% CI 0.58-0.88; $p < 0.01$) [118]. These data demonstrated role of immunotherapy as new treatment option for patients with advanced NSClC. Its role in NSCLC patient with BMs is currently under active investigation. Further phase III clinical trials are needed to evaluate existing options and develop new agents that can effectively cross the blood brain barrier.

REFERENCES

[1] Allemani C; Weir HK; Carreira H et al., Global surveillance of cancer survival 1995-2009: analysis of individual data for 25 676 887 patients from 279 population-based registries in 67 countries (CONCORD-2). *Lancet,* 2015 Mar 14; 385 (9972),977-1010.

[2] Schuette W. Treatment of brain metastases from lung cancer: chemotherapy. *Lung Cancer,* 2004 Aug; 45 Suppl 2, S253–7.

[3] Langer CJ; Mehta MP. Current management of brain metastases, with a focus on systemic options. *J Clin Oncol*, 2005 Sep 1; 23 (25),6207–6219.

[4] Coate LE; John T; Tsao M-S et al., Molecular predictive and prognostic markers in non-small-cell lung cancer. *Lancet Oncol*,2009 Oct; 10(10),1001–1010.

[5] Zhang I; Zaorsky NG; Palmer JD et al., Targeting brain metastases in ALK-rearranged non-small-cell lung cancer. *Lancet Oncol*, 2015 Oct;16(13):,e510-e521.

[6] Berger LA; Riesenberg H; Bokemeyer C et al., CNS metastases in nonsmall-cell lung cancer: current role of EGFR-TKI therapy and future perspectives. *Lung Cancer*, 2013 Jun;80,242–248.

[7] Dempke WC; Edvardsen K; Lu S et al., Brain Metastases in NSCLC - are TKIs Changing the Treatment Strategy? *Anticancer Res,* 2015 Nov;35(11),5797-5806.

[8] Shepherd FA; Pereira J; Ciuleanu TE et al., A randomized placebo-controlled trial of erlotinib in patients with advanced non-small cell lung cancer (NSCLC) following failure of 1st line or 2nd line chemotherapy. *J Clin Oncol,* 2004;22(suppl 14),12.

[9] Lynch TJ; Bell DW; Sordella R et al., Activating mutations in the epidermal growth factor receptor underlying responsiveness of non-small-cell lung cancer to gefitinib. *N Engl J Med*, 2004 May 20;350(21),2129–2139.

[10] Paez JG; Janne PA; Lee JC; et al., EGFR mutations in lung cancer: correlation with clinical response to gefitinib therapy. *Science*, 2004 Jun 4;304,1497–1500.

[11] Pao W; Miller V; Zakowski M et al., EGF receptor gene mutations are common in lung cancers from "never smokers" and are associated with sensitivity of tumors to gefitinib and erlotinib. *Proc Natl Acad Sci USA*, 2004 Sep 7;101(36),13306–13311.

[12] U.S. Food and Drug Administration. IRESSA® (ZD1839, gefitinib) Tablets. Oncologic Drugs Advisory Committee (ODAC) Meeting Briefing Document, March 4, 2005. Available at http://www.fda.gov/

[13] ohrms/dockets/ac/05/briefing/2005-4095B2_01_01-AstraZeneca-Iressa.pdf. Accessed July 12, 2005.

[14] Neville K; Parise RA; Lee JC et al., Plasma and cerebrospinal fluid pharmacokinetics of imatinib after administration to nonhuman primates. *Clin Cancer Res*, 2004 Apr 1; 10(7), 2525-2529.

[15] Togashi Y; Masago K; Fukudo M et al., Cerebrospinal fluid concentration of erlotinib and its active metabolite OSI-420 in patients with central nervous system metastases of non-small cell lung cancer. J *Thorac Oncol*, 2010 Jul; 5(7),950–955.

[16] Anderson C; Astrup J; Gyldensted C. Quantitation of peritumoural oedema and the effect of steroids using NMR-relaxation time imaging and blood-brain barrier analysis. *Acta Neurochir Suppl* (Wien), 1994; 60, 413-415.

[17] Cohen M; Johnson JR; Chen YF et al., FDA drug approval summary: erlotinib (Tarceva®) Tablets. The Oncologist, 2005 Aug;10(7),461–466.

[18] Thatcher N; Chang A; Parikh P et al., Results of a phase III placebo-controlled study (ISEL) of gefitinib (IRESSA) plus best supportive care (BSC) in patients with advanced non-small-cell lung cancer (NSCLC) who had received 1 or 2 prior chemotherapy regimens. Proc Am Assoc Cancer Res, 2005; Late Breaking Session: LB-6.

[19] Schuler M; Wu YL; Hirsh V et al., First-line afatinib versus chemotherapy in patients with non-small cell lung cancer and common epidermal growth factor receptor gene mutations and brain metastases. *J Thorac Oncol*, 2015 Jan; 10(1),156–163.

[20] Christensen JG; Zou HY; Arango ME et al., Cytoreductive antitumor activity of PF-2341066, a novel inhibitor of anaplastic lymphoma kinase and c-Met, in experimental models of anaplastic large-cell lymphoma. *Mol Cancer Ther*, 2007 Dec;6,3314-3322.

[21] Zou HY, Li Q, Lee JH, et al., An orally available small-molecule inhibitor of c-Met, PF-2341066, exhibits cytoreductive antitumor efficacy through antiproliferative and antiangiogenic mechanisms. *Cancer Res*, 2007 May 1;67(9),4408-4417.

[22] McDermott U; Iafrate AJ; Gray NS et al., Genomic alterations of anaplastic lymphoma kinase may sensitize tumors to anaplastic lymphoma kinase inhibitors. *Cancer Res*, 2008 May 1;68(9), 3389-3395.

[23] Shaw AT; Kim DW; Nakagawa K et al., crizotinib versus chemotherapy in advanced ALK-positive lung cancer. *N Engl J Med*, 2013 Jun 20; 368(25),2385-2394.

[24] Solomon BJ; Mok T; Kim DW et.al. First-line crizotinib versus chemotherapy in ALK-positive lung cancer. *N Engl J Med*, 2014 Dec 4; 371(23), 2167-2177.

[25] Costa DB; Kobayashi S; Pandya SS et al., CSF concentration of the anaplastic lymphoma kinase inhibitor crizotinib. *J Clin Oncol*, 2011 May 20; 29(20), e443-445.

[26] Costa DB; Shaw AT; Ou SH et al., Clinical Experience With Crizotinib in Patients With Advanced ALK-Rearranged Non-Small-Cell Lung Cancer and Brain Metastases. *J Clin Oncol*, 2015 Jun 10;33(17),1881-1888.

[27] Ou SH; Jänne PA; Bartlett CH et al., Clinical benefit of continuing ALK inhibition with crizotinib beyond initial disease progression in patients with advanced ALK-positive NSCLC. *Ann Oncol*, 2014 Feb;25(2),415-422.

[28] Weickhardt AJ; Scheier B; Burke JM et al., Local ablative therapy of oligoprogressive disease prolongs disease control by tyrosine kinase inhibitors in oncogene-addicted non-small-cell lung cancer. *J Thorac Oncol,* 2012 Dec;7(12),1807-1814.

[29] Seto T; Kiura K; Nishio M et al., CH5424802 (RO5424802) for patients with ALK-rearranged advanced non-small-cell lung cancer (AF-001JP study): a single-arm, open-label, phase 1-2 study. *Lancet Oncol*, 2013 Jun;14(7),590-598.

[30] Shaw AT; Kim DW; Mehra R et al., Ceritinib in ALK-rearranged non-small-cell lung cancer. *N Engl J Med*, 2014 Jun 26;370(26),1189-1197.

[31] Friboulet L; Li N; Katayama R et al., The ALK inhibitor ceritinib overcomes crizotinib resistance in non-small cell lung cancer. *Cancer Discov,* 2014 Jun;4(6),662-673.

[32] Marsilje TH; Pei W; Chen B et al., Synthesis, structure-activity relationships, and in vivo efficacy of the novel potent and selective anaplastic lymphoma kinase (ALK) inhibitor 5-chloro-N2-(2-isopropoxy-5-methyl-4-(piperidin-4-yl)phenyl)-N4-(2-(isopropylsulfonyl)phenyl)pyrimidine-2,4-diamine (LDK378) currently in phase 1 and phase 2 clinical trials. *J Med Chem*, 2013 Jul 25;56(14),5675-5690.

[33] Kim DW; Mehra R; Tan DS et al. Activity and safety of ceritinib in patients with ALK-rearranged non-small-cell lung cancer (ASCEND-1): updated results from the multicenter, open-label, phase 1 trial. *Lancet Oncol*, 2016 Apr; 17(4): 452-463.

[34] Zou HY; Friboulet L; Kodack DP et al., PF-06463922, an aLK/ ROS1 inhibitor, overcomes resistance to first and second generation inhibitors in preclinical models. *Cancer Cell*, 2015 Jul 13; 28(1): 70-81.

[35] Tamura T; T. Nakagawa K; et al., Updated data of a phase I/II study (AF-001JP) of alectinib, a CNS-penetrant, highly selective ALK inhibitor in ALK-rearranged advanced NSCLC. *Int J Radiant Oncol Biol Phys*, 2014; 90 (suppl): S6 abstr 10.

[36] Gainor JF; Sherman CA; Willoughby K et al., Alectinib salvages CNS relapses in ALK-positive lung cancer patients previously treated with crizotinib and ceritinib. *J Thorac Oncol*, 2015 Feb;10(2), 232-36.

[37] Sharma SV; Bell DW; Settleman J et al., Epidermal growth factor receptor mutations in lung cancer. *Nat Rev Cancer*, 2007 Mar;7(3),169–181

[38] Heon S; Yeap BY; Britt GJ et al., Development of central nervous system metastases in patients with advanced non-small cell lung cancer and somatic EGFR mutations treated with gefitinib or erlotinib. Clin *Cancer Res,* 2010 Dec 1;16(23),5873–5882.

[39] Omuro AM; Kris MG; Miller VA et al., High incidence of disease recurrence in the brain and leptomeninges in patients with nonsmall cell lung carcinoma after response to gefitinib. *Cancer*, 2005 Jun 1;103(11), 2344–2348.

[40] Eichler AF; Kahle KT; Wang DL et al., EGFR mutation status and survival after diagnosis of brain metastasis in nonsmall cell lung cancer. *Neuro Oncol*, 2010 Nov;12(11),1193–1199.

[41] Clarke JL; Pao W; Wu N et al., High dose weekly erlotinib achieves therapeutic concentrations in CSF and is effective in leptomeningeal metastases from epidermal growth factor receptor mutant lung cancer. *J Neurooncol*, 2010 Sep;99(2),283–286.

[42] Jackman DM; Holmes AJ; Lindeman N et al., Response and resistance in a non-small-cell lung cancer patient with an epidermal growth factor receptor mutation and leptomeningeal metastases treated with highdose gefitinib. *J Clin Oncol*, 2006 Sep 20;24(27),4517–4520.

[43] Christian G; Oxnard GR; Kris MG et al., "Pulsatile" high-dose weekly erlotinib for CNS metastases from EGFR mutant non-small cell lung cancer. *Neuro Oncol*, 2011 Dec;13(12),1364–1369.

[44] Engelman JA; Janne PA; Mermel C et al., ErbB-3 mediates phosphoinositide 3-kinase activity in gefitinibsensitive non-small cell lung cancer cell lines. *Proc Natl Acad Sci*, 2005 Mar 8;102(10),3788–3793.

[45] Baselga J; Rischin D; Ranson M et al., Phase I safety, pharmacokinetic, pharmacodynamic trial of ZD1839, a selective oral epidermal growth factor receptor tyrosine kinase inhibitor. *J Clin Oncol*, 2002 Nov 1; 20(21), 4292–4302.

[46] Clarke JL; Pao W; Wu N et al., High dose weekly erlotinib achieves therapeutic concentrations in CSF and is effective in leptomeningeal metastases from epidermal growth factor receptor mutant lung cancer. *J Neurooncol*, 2010 Sep; 99(2):283–286.

[47] Jackman DM; Cioffredi LA; Jocobs L et al. ,A Phase I trial of high dose gefitinib for patients with leptomeningeal metastases from non-small cell lung cancer. *Oncotarget*, 2015 Feb; 6(6), 4527-4536.

[48] Hoffknecht P; Tufman A; Wehler T et al., Efficacy of the irreversible ErbB family blocker afatinib in epidermal growth factor receptor (EGFR) tyrosine kinase inhibitor (TKI)-pretreated non-small-cell lung cancer patients with brain metastases or leptomeningeal disease. *J Thorac Oncol*, 2015 Jan; 10(1), 156-163.

[49] Li D; Ambrogio L; Shimamura T et al., BIBW2992, an irreversible EGFR/HER2 inhibitor highly effective in preclinical lung cancer models. *Oncogene,* 2008 Aug 7;27(34): 4702–4711.

[50] Cross DAE; Ashton SE; Ghiorghiu S et al., AZD9291, an irreversible EGFR TKI, overcomes T790M-mediated resistance to EGFR inhibitors in lung cancer. *Cancer Discovery,* 2014 Sep;4(9),1146–1161.

[51] Ahn MJ et al., AZD9291 activity in patients with EGFR-mutant advanced non-small cell lung cancer (NSCLC) and brain metastases: data from phase II studies. *Eur J Cancer*,2015; 51. Abstract #3083.

[52] Kim DW; Mehra R; Tan DSW et al., Ceritinib in advanced anaplastic lymphoma kinase (ALK) - rearranged (ALK+) non-small cell lung cancer (NSCLC): results of the ASCEND-1 trial. *J Clin Oncol*, 2014; 32(5s), 422s.

[53] Gainor JF; Sherman CA; Willoughby K et al., Alectinib salvages CNS relapses in ALK-positive lung cancer patients previously treated with crizotinib and ceritinib. *J Thorac Oncol*, 2015 Feb;10(2),232-236.

[54] Gadgeel SM; gandhi L; Riely GJ et al., Safety and activity of alectinib against systemic disease and brain metastases in patients with crizotinib-resistant ALD-rearranged non-small-cell lunga cancer (AF-002JG): results from the dose-finding portion of a phase ½ study. *Lancet Oncol*, 2014 Sep; 15(10):1119-1128.

[55] Giaccone G. Epidermal growth factor receptor inhibitors in the treatment of non-small-cell lung cancer. *J Clin Onco*, 2005 May 10;23(14),3235–3242.

[56] Kwak EL; Bang YJ; Camidge DR et al., Anaplastic lymphoma kinase inhibition in non-small-cell lung cancer. *N Engl J Med*, 2010 Oct 28;363(18),1693–1703.

[57] Ding L; Getz G; Wheeler DA et al., Somatic mutations affect key pathways in lung adenocarcinoma. *Nature,* 2008 Oct 23;455(7216),1069–1075.

[58] Tsuta K; Kohno T; Yoshida A et al., RET-rearranged non-small-cell lung carcinoma: a clinicopathological and molecular analysis. *Br J Cancer,* 2014 Mar 18;110(6),1571–1578.

[59] Yu HA; Arcila ME; Rekhtman N et al., Analysis of tumor specimens at the time of acquired resistance to EGFR-TKI therapy in 155 patients with EGFR-mutant lung cancers. *Clin Cancer Res*, 2013 Apr 15;19(8), 2240–2247.

[60] Khosravi-Far R; Der CJ. The Ras signal transduction pathway. Cancer Metastasis Rev, 1994 Mar;1351. Biankin AV, Waddell N, Kassahn KS, et al., Australian Pancreatic Cancer Genome Initiative. Pancreatic cancer genomes reveal aberrations in axon guidance pathway genes. *Nature*, 2012 Nov 15;491(7424), 399–405.

[61] Cancer Genome Atlas Research Network. Comprehensive molecular profiling of lung adenocarcinoma. *Nature,* 2014 Jul 31;511(7511),543–550.

[62] Cancer Genome Atlas Research Network. Comprehensive genomic characterization of squamous cell lung cancers. *Nature,* 2012 Sep 27;489(7417),519–525.

[63] Robinson SD; O'Shaughnessy JA; Cowey CL et al., BRAF V600E-mutated lung adenocarcinoma with metastases to the brain responding to treatment with vemurafenib. *Lung Cancer*, 2014 Aug;85(2),326–330.

[64] Turner N; Grose R. Fibroblast growth factor signalling: from development to cancer. *Nat Rev Cancer*, 2010 Feb;10(2),116–129.

[65] Weiss J; Sos ML; Seidel D et al., Frequent and focal FGFR1 amplification associates with therapeutically tractable FGFR1 dependency in squamous cell lung cancer. *Sci Transl Med*, 2010 Dec 15;2(62),62ra93.

[66] Bremnes RM; Camps C; Sirera R. Angiogenesis in non-small cell lung cancer: the prognostic impact of neoangiogenesis and the cytokines VEGF and bFGF in tumours and blood. *Lung Cancer*, 2006 Feb;51(2):143–158.

[67] Iwasaki A; Kuwahara M; Yoshinaga Y et al., Basic fibroblast growth factor (bFGF) and vascular endothelial growth factor (VEGF) levels, as prognostic indicators in NSCLC. *Eur J Cardiothorac Surg*, 2004 Mar;25(3),443–448.

[68] Gavine PR; Mooney L; Kilgour E et al., AZD4547: an orally bioavailable, potent, and selective inhibitor of the fibroblast growth factor receptor tyrosine kinase family. *Cancer Res*, 2012 Apr 15;72(8),2045–2056.

[69] Zito CR; Jilaveanu LB; Anagnostou V et al., Multi-level targeting of the phosphatidylinositol-3-kinase pathway in non-small cell lung cancer cells. *PLoS One*,2012;7(2):e31331.

[70] Cairncross JG; Kim JH; Posner JB. Radiation therapy for brain metastases. *Ann Neurol*, 1980; 7(6), 529-542.

[71] Chatani M; Teshima T; Hata K et al., Whole brain irradiation for metastases from lung carcinoma: A clinical investigation. *Acta Radiol Oncol,* 1985 Jul-Aug; 24(4),311-314.

[72] Hoskin PJ; Crow J; Ford HT. The influence of extent and local management on the outcome of radiotherapy for brain metastatses. *Int J Radiat Onco Biol Phys*,1990 Jul; 19(1),111-115.

[73] Lin X; DeAngelis LM. Treatment of Brain Metastases. *J Clin Oncol*, 2015 Oct 20; 33(30), 3475-3484.

[74] Antoniou D; Kyprianou K; Stathopoulos GP et al., Response to radiotherapy in brain metastases and survival of patients with non-small cell lung cancer. *Oncol Rep*, 2005 Sep; 14(3), 733-736.

[75] Langley RE; Stephens RJ; Nankivell M et al., Interim data from the Medical Research Council QUARTZ Trial: does whole brain radiotherapy affect the survival and quality of life of patients with brain metastases from non-small cell lung cancer? *Clin Onco*(R Coll Radiol), 2013 Mar; 25(3),e23-30.

[76] Tsao MN; Lloyd N; Wong RK et al., Whole brain radiotherapy for the treatment of newly diagnosed multiple brain metastases. Cochrane *Database Syst Rev*,2012 Apr 18; 4,CD003869.

[77] Young DF; Posner JB; Chu F et al., Rapid-course radiation therapy of cerebral metastases: Results and complications. *Cancer,* 1974 Oct; 34(4),1069-1076.

[78] Meyers CA; Smith JA; Bezjak A et al., Neurocognitive function and progression in patients with brain metastases treated with whole-brain radiation and motexafin gadolinium: results of a randomized phase III trial. *J Clin Oncol*, 2004 Jan 1; 22(1), 157-165.

[79] Mehta MP; Shapiro WR; Phan SC et al., Motexafin gadolinium combined with prompt whole brain radiotherapy prolongs time to neurologic progression in non-small-cell lung cancer patients with brain metastases: results of a phase III trial. *Int J Radiat Oncol Biol Phys*, 2009 Mar 15; 73(4),1069–1076.

[80] Mehta MP; Rodrigus P; Terhaard CH et al., Survival and neurologic outcomes in a randomized trial of motexafin gadolinium and whole-brain radiation therapy in brain metastases. *J Clin Oncol*, 2003 Jul 1; 21(13), 2529–36.

[81] Scott C; Suh J; Stea B et al., Improved survival, quality of life, and quality-adjusted survival in breast cancer patients treated with efaproxiral (Efaproxyn) plus whole-brain radiation therapy for brain metastases. *Am J Clin Oncol*, 2007 Dec; 30(6),580–587.

[82] Suh JH; Stea B; Nabid A et al., Phase III study of efaproxiral as an adjunct to whole-brain radiation therapy for brain metastases. *J Clin Oncol,* 2006 Jan 1;24(1),106–114.

[83] DeAngelis LM; Currie VE; Kim JH et al.,The combined use of radiation therapy and lonidamine in the treatment of brain metastases. *J Neurooncol,* 1989 Sep; 7(3),241-247.

[84] Eyre HJ; Ohlsen JD; Frank J et al., Randomized trial of radiotherapy versus radiotherapy plus metronidazole for the treatment metastatic cancer to brain: A Southwest Oncology Group study. *J Neurooncol,* 1984; 2(4),325-330.

[85] Komarnicky LT; Phillips TL; Martz K et al., A randomized phase III protocol for the evaluation of misonidazole combined with radiation in the treat- ment of patients with brain metastases (RTOG- 7916). *Int J Radiat Oncol Biol Phys*, 1991 Jan; 20(1),53-58.

[86] Phillips TL; Scott CB; Leibel SA et al., Results of a randomized comparison of radiotherapy and bromodeoxyuridine with radiotherapy alone for brain metastases: Report of RTOG trial 89-05. *Int J Radiat Oncol Biol Phys*, 1995 Sep 30; 33,339-348.

[87] Gondi V; Tome WA; Mehta MP. Why avoid the hippocampus? A comprehensive review. *Radiother Oncol*, 2010 Dec; 97(3), 370–376.

[88] Gondi V; Pugh SL; Tome WA et al., Preservation of mmemory with conformal avoidence of the hippocampal neural stem-cell compartment during whole-brain radiotherapy for brain metastases (RTOC 0933): a phase II multi-institutional trial. *J Clin Oncol*, 2014 Dec 1;32(34),3810-3816.

[89] Jatoi A; Kahanic SP; Frytak S et al., Donepezil and vitamin E for preventing cognitive dysfunction in small cell lung cancer patients: Preliminary results and suggestions for future study designs. *Support Care Cancer*, 2005 Jan; 13(1),66-69.

[90] Brown PD; Pugh S; Laack NN et al., Memantine for the prevention of cognitive dysfunction in patients receiving whole-brain radiotherapy: A randomized, double-blind, placebo-controlled trial. *Neuro Oncol*, 2013 Oct;15(10),1429-1437.

[91] Akimoto T; Hunter NR; Buchmiller L et al., Inverse relationship between epidermal growth factor receptor expression and radiocurability of murine carcinomas. *Clin Cancer Res*,1999 Oct; 5(10),2884-2890.

[92] Chinnaiyan P; Huang S; Vallabhaneni Get al., Mechanisms of enhanced radiation response following epidermal growth factor receptor signaling inhibition by erlotinib (Tarceva). *Cancer Res*, 2005 Apr 15; 65(8):3328-3335.

[93] Welsh JW; Komaki R; Amimi A et al., Phase II trial of erlotinib plus concurrent whole-brain radiation therapy for patients with brain metastasess from non-small-cell lung cancer. *J Clin Oncol*, 2013 Mar 1;31(7),895-902.

[94] Lu Y; Fan Y. Combined action of EGFR tyrosine kinase inhibitors and whole-brain radiotherapy on EGFR-mutated non-small-cell lung cancer patients with brain metastasis. *Onco Targets Ther*, 2016 Mar 9;9,1135-1143.

[95] Fan Y; Huang Z; Fang L et al., A phase II study of icotinib and whole-brain radiotherapy in Chinese patients with brain metastasis from non-small lung cancer. *Cancer Chemother Pharmacol*, 2015 Sep;76(3), 517-523.

[96] Zheng MH; Sun HT; Xu JG et al., Combining whole-brain radiotherapy with Gefitinib/Erlotinib for brain metastases from non-small-cell lung cancer: a meta-analysis. *Biomed Res Int*, 2016;2016,5807346.

[97] Kondziolka D; Patel A; Lunsford LD et al., Stereotactic radiosurgery plus whole brain radiotherapy versus radiotherapy alone for patients with multiple brain metastases. *Int J Radiat Oncol Biol Phys*, 1999 Sep 1;45(2),427-434.

[98] Andrew DW; Scott CB; Sperduto PW et al., Whole brain radiation therapy with or without stereotactic radio surgery boost for patients with one to three brain metastases: phase III results of the RTOG 9508 Randomised trial. *Lancet,* 2004 May 22; 363(9422),1665-1672.

[99] Aoyama H; Shirato H; Tago M et al., Stereotactic radiosurgery plus whole-radiation therapy vs stereotactic radiosurgery alone for treatment of brain metastases: a randomized controlled trial. *JAMA*, 2006 Jun 7; 295(21),2483-91.

[100] Kocher M; Soffietti R; Abaciogu U et al., Adjuvant whole-brain radiotherapy vs observation after radio surgery or surgical resection of one to three cerebral metastases: results of the EORTC 22952-26001 study. *J Clin Oncol*, 2011 Jan 10;29(2),134-141.

[101] 93. Aoyama H; Tago M; Shirato H et al., Stereotactic radiosurgery with or without whole-brain radiotherapy for brain metastases: secondary analysis of the JROSG 99-1 randomized clinical trial. *JAMA Oncol*, 2015 Jul; 1(4),457-464.

[102] Chang EL; Wefel JS; Hess KR et al. Neurocognition in patients with brain metastases treated with radiosurgery or radiosurgery plus whole-brain irradiation: a randomised controlled trial. *Lancet Oncol*, 2009 Nov; 10(11),1037–1044.

[103] Hall MD; McGee JL; McGee MC et al., Cost-effectiveness of stereotactic radiosurgery with and without whole-brain radiotherapy for the treat- ment of newly diagnosed brain metastases. *J Neurosurg,* 2014 Dec;121, 84-90.

[104] Sahgal A; Aoyama H; Kocher M et al., Phase 3 trials of stereotactic radiosurgery with or without whole-brain radiation therapy for 1 to 4 brain metastases: individual patient data meta-analysis. *Int J Radiat Oncol Biol Phys,* 2015 Mar 15;91(4),710–717.

[105] Serizawa T; Hirai T; Nagano O et al., Gamma knife surgery for 1-10 brain metastases without prophylactic whole- brain radiation therapy: analysis of cases meeting the Japanese prospective multi-institute study (JLGK0901) inclusion criteria. *J Neurooncol*, 2010 Jul;98(2),163–167.

[106] Yamamoto M; Serizawa T; Shuto T et al., Stereotactic radiosurgery for patients with multiple brain metastases (JLGK0901): A multi-institutional prospective observational study. *Lancet Oncol*, 2014 Apr; 15,387-395.

[107] Patchell RA; Tibbs PA; Walsh JW et al., A randomized trial of surgery in the treatment of single metastases to the *brain. N Engl J* Med, 1990 Feb 22; 322,494-500.

[108] Vecht CJ; Haaxma-Reiche H; Noordijk EM et al., Treatment of single brain metastasis: Radiother- apy alone or combined with neurosurgery? *Ann Neurol*, 1993 Jun; 33, 583-590.

[109] 104. Mintz AH; Kestle J; Rathbone MP et al. A randomized trial to assess the efficacy of surgery in addition to radiotherapy in patients with a single cerebral metastasis. *Cancer,*1996 Oct 1; 78,1470-1476.

[110] Patchell RA; Tibbs PA; Regine WF et al. Postoperative radiotherapy in the treatment of single metastases to the brain: A randomized trial. *JAMA,*1998 Nov 4; 280,1485-1489.

[111] Schoggl A; Kitz K; Reddy M et al., Defining the role of stereotactic radiosurgery versus microsurgery in the treatment of single brain metastases. *Acta Neurochir*, 2000;142(6),621–626.

[112] Wang TJ; Saad S; Qureshi YH et al., Outcomes of gamma knife radiosurgery, bi-modality and tri-modality treatment regimens for patients with one or multiple brain metastases: the Columbia University Medical Center experience. *J Neurooncol*, 2015 Apr;122(2), 339–408.

[113] Auchter RM; Lamond JP; Alexander E et al., A multiinstitutional outcome and prognostic factor analysis of radiosurgery for resectable single brain metastasis. *Int J Radiat Oncol Biol Phys*, 1996 Apr 1; 35(1), 27–35.

[114] Qin H; Wang C; Jiang Y et al., Patients with single brain metastasis from non-small cell lung cancer equally benefit from stereotactic radiosurgery and surgery: a systematic review. *Med Sci Monit*, 2015 Jan 12; 21,144–152.

[115] NCCN guidelines version 4.2016 Non-Small Cell Lung Cancer. http://www.nccn.org/professionals/physician_gls/f_guidelines.asp#site.

[116] Porta R; Sánchez-Torres JM; Paz-Ares L et al., Brain metastases from lung cancer responding to erlotinib: the importance of EGFR mutation. *Eur Respir J*, 2011;37(3),624.

[117] Pochesci A; Passaro A; Catania C et al., Immunotherapy in non-small cell lung cancer: evolution of knowledge and clinic advances. *Recent Prog Med*, 2016 Apr; 107(4), 186-192.

[118] Brahmer J; Reckamp KL; Baas P et al., Nivolumab versus docetaxel in advanced squamous-cell non-small cell lung cancer. *N Engl J Med*, 2015 Jul 9; 373(2): 123-135.

[119] Borghaei H; Paz-Ares L; Horn L et al., Nivolumab versus docetaxel in advenced nonsquamous non-small cell lung cancer. *N Engl J Med*, 2015 Oct 22; 373(17),1627-1639.

[120] Herbst RS; Baas P; Kim DW et al., Pembrolizumab versus docetaxel for previously treated, PD-L1-positive advanced non-small-cell lung cancer (KEYNOTE-010): a randomized controlled trial. *Lacet,* 2016 Apr 9; 387(10027), 1540-1550.

In: Horizons in Cancer Research. Volume 63 ISBN: 978-1-53610-013-6
Editor: Hiroto S. Watanabe

Chapter 2

POSITIVE EFFECT OF MICROSCOPIC COMPLETE RESECTION ON CONTROLLING THE LOCAL RECURRENCE OF A SINGLE BRAIN METASTASIS

Ji Hwan Jang, MD and Young Zoon Kim, MD, PhD
Division of Neurooncology and Department of Neurosurgery
Sungkyunkwan University School of Medicine, Samsung Changwon Hospital, Changwon, Gyeongsangnam-do, Korea

ABSTRACT

Background; The influence on therapeutic outcome of the wide surgical resection of brain metastasis (BM) including tumor cells microscopically infiltrating adjacent brain parenchyma with confirming clean surgical margin by intraoperative margin biopsy is not known. This study was carried out to clarify the therapeutic impact of such resections.

Material and Methods; From June 2002 to December 2014, 90 patients (66 males and 24 females; mean age: 56.7 years) underwent surgical resection for BM. We undertook microscopic complete resection, including microscopic infiltrative tumor cells adjacent brain parenchyma, with confirming a pathologically clean surgical margin during surgery for the BMs located in a non-eloquent area in 47 patients (Group A), but in 43 patients, we undertook gross complete resection without removal of neighboring brain parenchyma due to their eloquent location (Group B).

The two groups were then compared in terms of survival, and local and distant recurrence.

Results; Mean follow-up duration was 18.6 month and 71 patients (78.9%) died during follow-up. Median survival times were 13.1 months in group A and 12.1 months in group B ($p = 0.309$). One-year and 2-year local recurrence rates were 21.2% and 25.8% in group A, and 65.2% and 65.2% in group B, respectively ($p = 0.000$). One-year and 2-year distant recurrence rates were 46.3% and 57.2% in group A, and 33.2% and 33.2% in group B, respectively ($p = 0.140$).

Conclusion; These results suggest that the wide surgical resection of BM including tumor cells infiltrating adjacent brain parenchyma with confirming clean surgical margin renders better local control.

Keywords: microscopic complete resection, brain metastasis, local control, survival, surgical resection, margin biopsy

INTRODUCTION

Although the true incidence is not known, it is estimated that 98,000 to 170,000 new cases of brain metastasis (BM) are diagnosed in the United States each years, with variations in the estimates of incidence and prevalence arising from differences in the method of assessment [8]. In the largest autopsy series to dates, Posner and Chernik examined the records of 2,375 cancer patients and found that central nervous system metastases occur in approximately 24% of patients with systemic cancer [15].

It has been accepted that some of the patients with BM could be treated with craniotomy for a palliative purpose, as usually combined with brain irradiation. As potential candidates for resection are considered, it is impossible to determine exactly who will benefit from surgical resection and post-resection treatment because of the limited survival time associated with BM. However, surgery for BM provides certain advantages over other therapeutic modalities [7]. First, the excision of a metastasis can immediately eliminate the effects of increased intracranial pressure and direct symptomatic effects on surrounding brain tissues. Second, surgery provides tissue for confirming a diagnosis of metastasis. Finally, surgery may establish a local cure or complete remission if all tumor cells can be removed.

The recent advances in microsurgical techniques, such as, navigation systems, intraoperative ultrasonography, and cortical mapping have promoted safe surgical resection, and this is particularly the case for single lesions, which account for 40~60% of all BMs [1,13]. And, modern imaging techniques are now able to locate and define smaller metastases that can be operated on earlier in their development.

However, despite the above advantages of surgery for BM, this approach has not been fully accepted because the tumor recurrence rate is high after BM resection [24]. Even if complete resection has been confirmed both by intraoperative evaluation and by immediate postoperative magnetic resonance (MR) imaging, increased patient survival inevitably increases the number of recurrences due to residual foci of microscopic and infiltrative tumor left behind at the time of surgery unexpectedly, particularly in eloquent areas of the brain, where attempts at achieving clean surgical margins increase the risk of neurological dysfunction. In fact, small nests and trabeculae of tumor cells can be seen at tumor borders to infiltrate adjacent nervous tissue under the microscope. However, this does not typically extend to more than 5 mm beyond the circumference of a solid tumor [22].

To reduce local recurrence, in the tumors located in non-eloquent areas, we undertook wide surgical resection of BMs including microscopic, infiltrative tumor cells adjacent brain parenchyma, and confirming clean surgical margin by intraoperative margin biopsy. However, when a tumor was located in an eloquent area, we undertook gross complete resection without additional removal of surrounding brain parenchyma. We evaluated the validity of wide surgical resection of BM including tumor cells microscopically infiltrating adjacent brain parenchyma by comparing these two patient groups in terms of local and distant recurrence rates, and overall survivals.

Material and Methods

Study Design

Between June 2002 and December 2014, 90 patients underwent craniotomy to remove a BM in our institute. Of these, 47 patients (group A) underwent wide surgical resection of BM including microscopic, infiltrative tumor cells adjacent brain parenchyma with a 5mm tumor free margin outside tumor capsules. The clean surgical margin was confirmed in each case by marginal biopsy during surgery. In brief, after identifying the gliotic pseudo-capsule surrounding the tumor through a transcortical or transsulcal approach, we attempted en bloc resection without rupturing the tumor compartment, if possible. After gross total removal of tumor, we resected additional surrounding brain tissue to at least a depth of 5mm until a pathologic free margin was confirmed. We defined the above pattern of surgical resection of BM as microscopic complete resection (MCR). Another group of 43 patients (Group B) underwent gross complete resection (GCR) of BM without additional resection of adjacent brain parenchyma due to their eloquent location. Methods of surgical resection of BM are illustrated schematically in Figure 1.

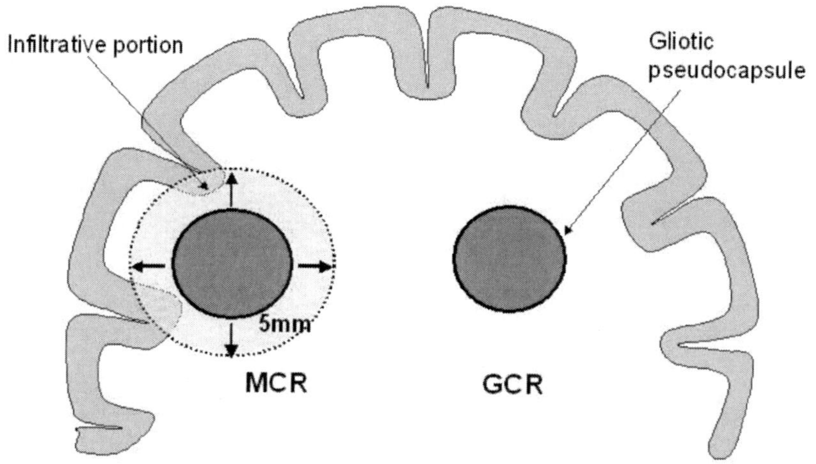

Figure 1. Methods of surgical resection in the group A and group B. In the group A, the microscopic complete resection (MCR) of brain metastasis included brain parenchyma which contained microscopic infiltrative tumor cells surrounding tumor and then clean surgical margin was confirmed by intraoperative margin biopsy. But, in the group B, gross complete resection (GCR) of brain metastasis was undergone without additional resection of adjust brain parenchyma due to their eloquent location.

Clinical Characteristics of Patients

Retrospective analysis of survival, local recurrence and distant recurrence in relation to the clinical variables that might affect them was performed. These variables included patient's age and gender, type of primary cancer, extracranial metastasis, status of primary cancer, Karnofsky Performance Scale (KPS) scores and recursive partitioning analysis (RPA) class.

According to the classification described by Gasper et al. [3], patients in RPA Class 1 were characterized by an age of <65 years, a KPS score of ≥70 and the absence of extracranial metastases, with good control of their systemic disease. The RPA Class 2 patients had a KPS score of ≥ 70, but may also had age ≥65 years, or had uncontrolled systemic disease or other systemic metastases. Patients in RPA Class 3 were those patients with a KPS of <70.

Features of brain metastasis

These variables included timing of metastasis, tumor size, tumor location, functional grade of lesion and method of tumor resection. Brain metastasis diagnosed <0 days from primary lesion diagnosis was considered synchronous, and brain metastasis diagnosed 60 days from the time of primary cancer diagnosis was defined as metachronous. Tumor size was determined as maximal orthogonal diameter and divided into <3 cm and ≥3 cm. The location of the tumor was categorized as either supratentorial or infratentorial. Using preoperative magnetic resonance imaging (MRI) study, each tumor was functionally graded relative to its location with respect to eloquent brain according to a scheme developed at M.D. Anderson Cancer Center [19]. Functional grade I tumors were located in non-eloquent brain (e.g., frontal or temporal polar lesion), grade II tumors in near eloquent brain (e.g., near motor or sensory cortex, near calcarine fissure, near speech center, near dentate nucleus, near brain stem or corpus callosum) and grade III tumors in eloquent brain (e.g., motor and sensory cortex, visual center, speech center, internal capsule, basal ganglia, hypothalamus, thalamus, brain stem and dentate nucleus).

Surgical Indications

Clinical indications included symptoms and signs of intracranial hypertension unresponsive to adequate medical therapy (e.g., corticosteroid and mannitol), intractable seizures, a reduced level of consciousness, progressive motor weakness, gait ataxia and aphasia. Neuro-imaging indications included lesion enlargement, hemorrhage, and a mass effect from edema unresponsive to maximal medical therapy.

Outcomes and Data Analysis

Survival times were defined from the date of surgical resection until death or until the last day of follow-up. Postsurgical imaging studies were reviewed for evidence of CNS recurrence. Local recurrences were defined as those within 2 cm of the initial tumor resection bed. Distant recurrences in the central nervous system (CNS) were defined as any of the following: >2 cm from the initial surgical site, on the contralateral side, in the posterior fossa, in the spinal cord, or in the cerebrospinal fluid. For patients who died, cause of death and date of death were recorded. The medical records of all patients were analyzed, including clinical history, operative and pathology reports, and radiological studies, and dates of death were confirmed for all patients that succumbed.

Statistical Analysis

Statistical analyses were performed using SSPS version 12.0 (SPSS Institute, Inc., Chicago, IL). Progression-free-survival (PFS) and overall survivals were estimated using Kaplan-Meier methods. The Log-rank test and Cox regression analysis were used to examine progression-free and overall survival. Variables found to be significantly associated with survival by univariate analyses were subject to multivariate analyses. The T-test and the Chi-square tests were used to compare the two groups in terms of baseline characteristics. Results were considered significant when p-values were less than 0.05.

RESULTS

Patient Populations

Table 1 summarizes patient characteristics. In group A, there were 35 men and 12 women of mean age 57.9 years (range: 14-84), and in group B, there were 31 men and 12 women of mean age 55.3 years (range: 12-77), when brain metastasis was diagnosed. The histological distribution of primary tumor types was follows: 66 non-small cell lung cancers, 3 small cell lung cancers, 7 colorectal cancers, 6 renal cell cancers, and 11 other systemic cancers.

Table 1. Clinical characteristics of the patients according to Group A and B

		Total (N = 90)	Group A (N = 47)	Group B (N = 43)	p value
Gender	male	66 (73.3%)	35 (74.5%)	31 (72.1%)	0.799
	female	24 (26.7%)	12 (25.5%)	12 (27.1%)	
Age	mean	56.66	57.87	55.33	0.335
	range	(12-84)	(14-84)	(12-77)	
	≥65	23 (25.6%)	16 (34.0%)	7 (16.3%)	0.054
	<65	67 (74.4%)	31 (66.0%)	36 (83.7%)	
Primary cancer	NSCLC*	63(70.0%)	34 (72.3%)	29 (67.4%)	0.612
	SCLC†	3 (3.3%)	3 (6.4%)	0 (0.0%)	
	colorectal	7 (7.8%)	3 (6.4%)	4 (9.3%)	
	kidney	6 (6.7%)	3 (6.4%)	3 (7.0%)	
	gynecology	3 (3.3%)	1 (2.1%)	2 (4.7%)	
	liver	3 (3.3%)	0 (0.0%)	1 (2.3%)	
	breast	2 (2.2%)	2 (4.3%)	2 (4.7%)	
	stomach	2 (2.2%)	1 (2.1%)	1 (2.3%)	
	others	1 (1.1%)	0 (0.0%)	1 (2.3%)	
Extracranial metastasis	presence	49 (54.4%)	28 (59.6%)	21 (48.8%)	0.307
	absence	41 (45.6%)	19 (40.4%)	22 (51.2%)	
Status of cancer	under-control	56 (62.2%)	29 (61.7%)	27 (62.8%)	0.915
	out-of-control	34 (37.8%)	18 (38.3%)	16 (37.2%)	
KPS‡ score	≥70	62 (68.9%)	39 (83.0%)	23 (53.5%)	*0.003*
	<70	28 (31.1%)	8 (17.0%)	20 (46.5%)	
RPA§ class	1	16 (17.8%)	10 (21.3%)	6 (14.0%)	*0.001*
	2	49 (54.4%)	32 (68.1%)	17 (39.5%)	
	3	25 (27.8%)	5 (10.6%)	20 (46.5%)	

NSCLC*; non-small cell lung cancer, SCLC†; small cell lung cancer, KPS‡; Karnofsky Performance Scale, RPA§; Recursive Partitioning Analysis

Table 2. Features of the brain metastasis according to Group A and B

		Total (N = 90)	Group A (N = 47)	Group B (N = 43)	p value
Timing of metastasis	synchronous	34 (37.8%)	22 (46.8%)	12 (27.9%)	0.065
	metachronous	56 (62.2%)	25 (53.2%)	31 (72.1%)	
Tumor size	<3cm	31 (34.4%)	12 (25.5%)	19 (44.2%)	0.063
	≥3cm	59 (65.6%)	35 (74.5%)	24 (55.8%)	
Tumor location	supratentorial	75 (83.3%)	37 (78.7%)	38 (88.4%)	0.220
	infratentorial	15 (16.7%)	10 (21.3%)	5 (11.6%)	
Functional grade	1	23 (25.6%)	22 (46.8%)	1 (2.3%)	*0.000*
	2	45 (50.0%)	18 (38.3%)	27 (62.8%)	
	3	22 (24.1%)	7 (14.9%)	15 (34.9%)	
Postoperative radiotherapy	yes	29 (32.2%)	4 (8.5%)	25 (58.1%)	*0.000*
	no	61 (67.8%)	43 (91.5%)	18 (41.9%)	

Forty-nine patients (54.4%) had extracranial metastases (28 (59.6%) in group A and 21 (48.8%) in group B). Fifty-six cancers (62.2%) lied under control but 28 cancers (37.8%) were progressing. Sixty-two patients (68.9%) had a Karnofsky Performance Scale (KPS) scores of ≥70 (39 (83.0%) in group A and 23 (53.5%) in group B). In group A, 10 patients (21.3%) were included in the RPA class I, 32 patients (68.1%) in RPA class II and 5 patients (10.6%) in RPA class III. And in group B, 6 patients (14.0%) were included in the RPA class I, 17 patients (39.5%) in the RPA class II, 20 patients (46.5%) in RPA class III.

No significant difference was observed between the two groups in terms of demographic parameters or features of patients. However, group A had higher KPS score ($p = 0.003$) and lower RPA class ($p = 0.001$) than group B.

Features of Brain Metastasis

Table 2 shows features of brain lesions. Fifty-six patients (25 in group A and 31 in group B) had metachronous development, whereas the others (22 in group A and 12 in group B) had synchronous development. Twenty-three tumors were included in the functional grade 1 (22 in group A and 1 in group

B), 45 in the functional grade 2 (18 in group A and 7 in group B) and 22 in the functional grade 3 (7 in group A and 15 in group B) ($p = 0.000$). Twenty-nine patients (4 (8.5%) in group A and 25 (58.1%) in group B) received radiotherapy after BM surgery ($p = 0.000$). In the features of brain metastasis, functional grade of tumor ($p = 0.000$) and postoperative radiotherapy ($p = 0.000$) had statistical differences between two groups.

Postoperative Follow-Up

No patients were lost during follow-up. The absence of residual enhancing lesions was confirmed by immediate postoperative MRI within 48 hours of surgery. All patients underwent a regular MRI study at one month after surgery and then 3 monthly or when clinically indicated. Overall median survival time (MST) for the all the patients was 12.4 (range: 3.2-56.8). In group A, MST was 13.1 months (range: 3.3-56.8) and in group B, 12.1 months (range: 3.2-47.8).

During follow-up period, seventy-one (78.9%) patients died (35 (74.5%) in group A and 36 (83.7%) in group B). Most of them succumbed to a systemic cause, i.e., progression of primary cancer or complication of primary disease. Four patients died from CNS problems; one patient succumbed to a massive hypertensive intracerebral hemorrhage in a location remote from the brain metastasis at 124 days after surgery and the other three patients did to meningeal carcinomatosis. Strictly speaking, the only three patients (3.3%) died from CNS origin.

Analysis of Survivals

Table 3 summarizes the survival analysis according to group A and B. The MST was calculated from the date of surgery for BM. In group A, MST was 13.1 months (range: 3.3-56.8) and in group B, 12.1 months (range: 3.2-47.8). One-year survival rate was 55.2% in group A and 50.6% in group B. Two-year survival rate was 25.6% in group A and 10.7% in group B. No statistical difference was observed in median survival, 1-year survival rate and 2-year survival rate ($p = 0.309$). Cox regression model analysis showed no superiority in Hazard ratio between two groups. Figure 2 showed the overall survival and the difference of survival between the two groups according to follow-up by using Kaplan-Meier survival curves.

Table 3. Survival analysis and 1-year and 2-year survival rates according to Group A and B

	Total (N = 90)	Group A (N = 47)	Group B (N = 43)
Mean survival (month)	18.6	21.1	14.6
Median survival (month)	12.4	13.1	12.1
Ranges (month)	3.2-56.8	3.3-56.8	3.2-47.8
1-year survival rate	52.9%	55.2%	50.6%
2-year survival rate	19.3%	25.6%	10.7%

Table 4. Clinical characteristics of the patients affecting survival in univariate and multivariate analysis (Cox regression model)

Factor		median survival (month)	univariate analysis (p value)	Hazard ratio (95% CI*)	multivariate analysis (p value)	Hazard ratio (95% CI)
Gender	male	9.1	*0.024*	1.77 (1.07, 2.91)	*0.013*	1.94 (1.15, 3.27)
	female	13.6				
Age	≥65 years	10.0	*0.033*	1.75 (1.04, 2.96)	*0.024*	1.89 (1.09, 3.28)
	<65 years	13.4				
Pathology	NSCLC†	11.8	0.083	1.54 (0.94, 2.50)	NA‡	
	non-NSCLC	13.6				
Extracranial metastasis	presence	11.7	0.066	1.56 (0.97, 2.50)	NA	
	absence	13.5				
Status of cancer	under-control	12.3	0.181	1.39 (0.86, 2.26)	NA	
	out-of-control	13.5				
KPS§ score	≥70	13.9	*0.003*	2.04 (1.26, 3.32)	*0.000*	12.76 (3.36, 46.43)
	<70	5.6				
Postoperative radiotherapy	yes	12.1	0.250	1.33 (0.82, 2.16)	0.994	1.00 (0.54, 1.87)
	no	12.4				

CI*; confidence interval, NSCLC†; non-small cell lung cancer, NA‡; not assessed, KPS§; Karnofsky Performance Scale

Table 5. Features of the brain metastasis affecting survival in univariate and multivariate analysis (Cox regression model)

Factor		median survival (month)	univariate analysis (month)	Hazard ratio (95% CI*)	multivariate analysis (month)	Hazard ratio (95% CI)
Timing of metastasis	synchronous	13.5	0.398	1.24 (0.76, 2.02)	NA†	
	metachronous	11.7				
Tumor size	<3cm	13.9	0.968	1.01 (0.62, 1.64)	NA	
	≥3cm	12.1				
Tumor locations	supratentorial	13.1	0.465	1.26 (0.68, 2.35)	NA	
	infratentorial	10.3				
Method of surgery	MCR‡	13.1	0.309	1.27 (0.80, 2.04)	0.776	1.09 (0.59, 2.01)
	GTR§	12.1				

CI*; confidence interval, NA†; not assessed, MCR‡; microscopic complete resection, GTR§; gross total resection

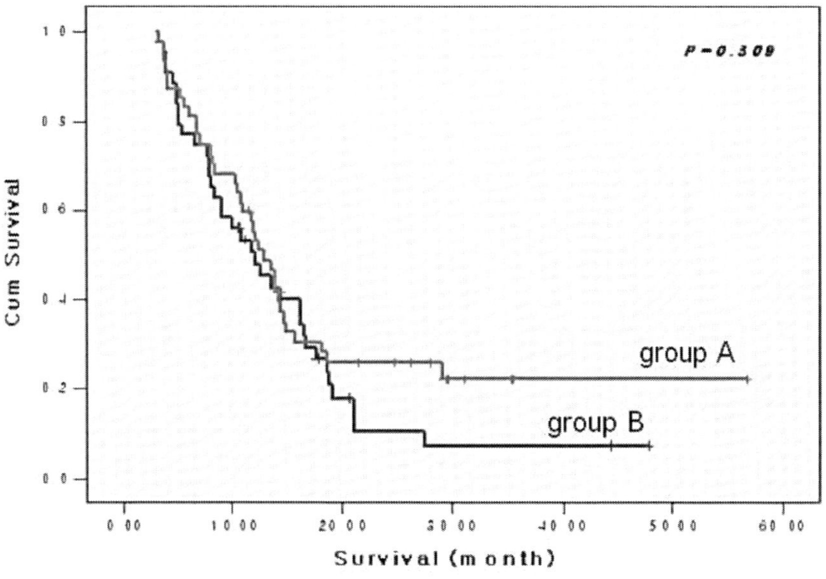

Figure 2. Actual survivals in the group A and the group B.

In addition to method of surgical resection of BM, we also searched for associations between other factors (e.g., gender, age, pathology, tumor stage, extracranial metastasis, status of primary tumor, KPS score, timing of metastasis, tumor size, location, functional grade and postoperative radiotherapy) and survival. The clinical variables of female gender, age <65 years, and KPS score of ≥70 were considered to experience better survival outcome, as were estimated by use of univariate and multivariate survival analysis (Table 4). But none of the factors of brain lesion had an association with survival (Table 5).

Local Recurrences

Table 6 shows patterns of local recurrence according to group A and B. Thirty-two patients (35.6%) had local recurrence; 9 patients (19.1%) in group A and 23 (53.5%) in group B (p = 0.000). In group A, 1-year and 2-year local recurrence rates were 21.2% and 25.8%, respectively and, in group B, 65.2% and 65.2%, respectively. In group A, median time-to-progression (TTP) was not reached at median period during follow-up, whereas, in group B, median TTP was 8.84 months. Actual PFS curves are presented in Figure 3.

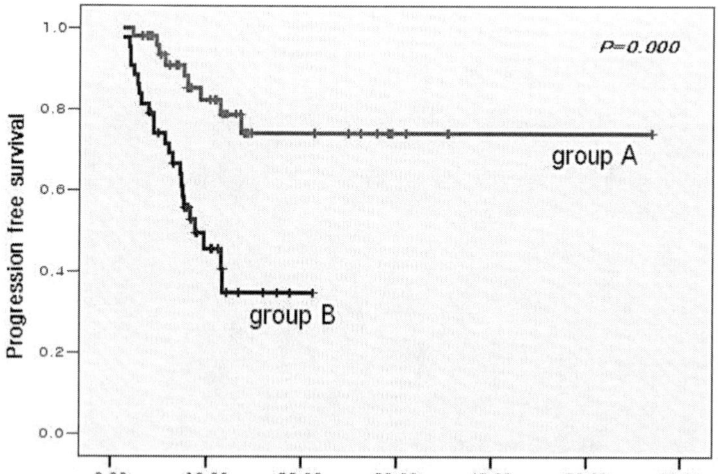

Figure 3. In terms of local recurrence, progression-free survival according to group A and B.

Table 6. Local recurrence analysis and 1-year and 2-year recurrence rates according to Group A and B

	Total (N = 90)	Group A (N = 47)	Group B (N = 43)
Number of patients	32 (35.6%)	9 (19.1%)	23 (53.5%)
Mean TTP* (month)	34.6	44.3	11.5
Median TTP (month)	NR†	NR	8.8
Ranges (month)	1.2-56.8	2.3-56.8	1.2-21.2
1-year recurrence rate	41.7%	21.2%	65.2%
2-year recurrence rate	44.5%	25.8%	65.2%

Table 7. Clinical characteristics of the patients affecting local recurrence in univariate and multivariate analysis (Cox regression model)q

Factor		median survival (month)	univariate analysis (p value)	Hazard ratio (95% CI*)	multivariate analysis (p value)	Hazard ratio (95% CI)
Gender	male	NR†	0.871	1.07 (0.48, 2.38)	NA‡	
	female	NR				
Age	≥65 years	NR	0.139	3.03 (0.78, 5.26)	NA	
	<65 years	NR				
Pathology	NSCLC§	NR	0.229	1.67 (0.72, 3.85)	NA	
	non-NSCLC	NR				
Extracranial metastasis	presence	NR	0.984	1.01 (0.48, 2.13)	NA	
	absence	NR				
Status of cancer	under-control	NR	0.685	1.16 (0.57, 2.34)	NA	
	out-of-control	NR				
KPS score	≥70	NR	*0.040*	2.97 (1.48, 5.95)	0.067	2.14 (1.03, 4.44)
	<70	8.3				
Postoperative radiotherapy	yes	NR	0.062	1.60 (0.86, 3.06)	0.182	1.28 (0.63, 2.18)
	no	11.6				

CI*; confidence interval, NR†; not reached at median value, NA‡; not assessed, NSCLC§; non-small cell lung cancer, KPS; Karnofsky Performance Scale

Table 8. Features of the brain metastasis affecting local recurrence in univariate and multivariate analysis (Cox regression model)

Factor		median survival (month)	univariate analysis (month)	Hazard ratio (95% CI*)	multivariate analysis (month)	Hazard ratio (95% CI)
Timing of metastasis	synchronous	NR[†]	0.134	1.79 (0.83, 3.87)	NA[‡]	
	metachronous	NR				
Tumor size	<3cm	NR	0.058	1.94 (0.97, 3.88)	NA	
	≥3cm	NR				
Tumor locations	supratentorial	NR	0.055	3.70 (0.88, 15.49)	NA	
	infratentorial	NR				
Method of surgery	MCR[§]	NR	*0.000*	3.84 (1.77, 8.32)	*0.007*	3.09 (1.37, 6.96)
	GTR□	11.6				

CI*; confidence interval, NR†; not reached at median value, NA‡; not assessed, MCR§; microscopic complete resection, GTR; gross total resection

By Cox regression analysis, the Hazard ratio of local recurrence for group B versus group A was 3.84 (95% Confidence Interval, 1.77-8.32; p = 0.000) in univariate analysis and 3.09 (95% Confidence Interval, 1.37-6.96; p = 0.007) in multivariate analysis. In addition to method of surgical resection of BM, we also examined association between other risk factors (e.g., gender, age, pathology, tumor stage, extracranial metastasis, status of primary tumor, KPS score, timing of metastasis, tumor size, location, functional grade and postoperative radiotherapy) and local recurrence. According to univariate analyses, KPS score was associated with local recurrence but not associated with local recurrence in multivariate analyses after multi-factor adjustment (Tables 7 and 8).

Distant Recurrences

Table 9 shows patterns of distant recurrence according to group A and B. Thirty-two patients (35.6%) had distant recurrences; 21 (44.7%) of 47 patients in group A and 11 (25.6%) of 43 patients in group B. Median TTP in group A was 20.3 months, but distant recurrence in group B, was not reached at median value during follow-up. Actual PFS curves are presented in Figure 4.

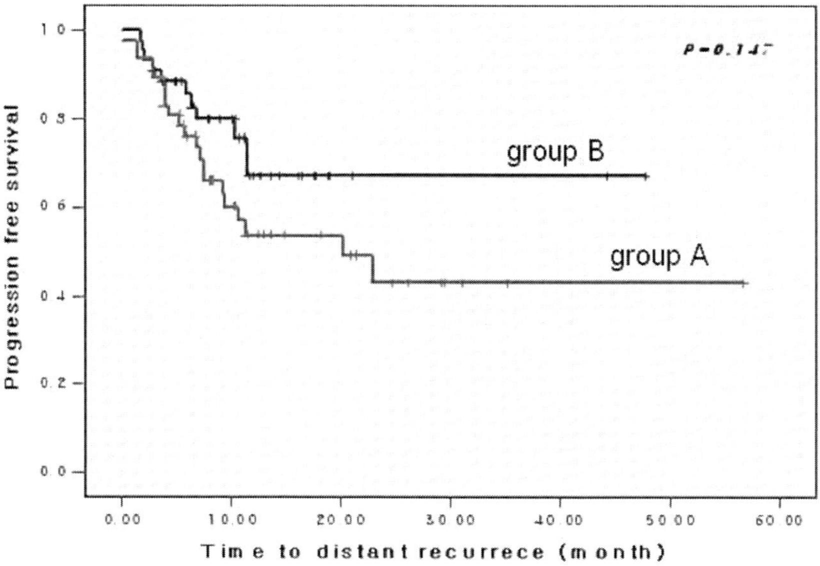

Figure 4. In terms of distant recurrence, progression- free survival according to group A and B.

Table 9. Distant recurrence analysis and 1-year and 2-year recurrence rates according to Group A and B

	Total (N = 90)	Group A (N = 47)	Group B (N = 43)
Number of patients	32 (35.6%)	21 (44.7%)	11 (25.6%)
Mean TTP* (month)	32.3	29.5	34.3
Median TTP (month)	NR†	20.3	NR
Ranges (month)	0.4-56.8	0.4-56.8	1.9-47.8
1-year recurrence rate	40.2%	46.3%	33.2%
2-year recurrence rate	49.8%	57.2%	33.2%

As shown in Table 11, no statistical difference in distant recurrence between two groups was found by Kaplan-Meier model and Cox regression analysis. And in Table 10, the Hazard ratio of distant recurrence for the patients under well-controlled primary cancer versus those with out-of-controlled primary cancer was 2.61 (95% Confidence Interval, 1.29-5.26; p = 0.005) in univariate analysis. Other factors affecting distant recurrences, such as, status of primary cancer and KPS score, were associated with distant recurrence in univariate analysis. But, in multivariate analysis, KPS score was not associated with distant recurrence after multi-factor adjustment.

Table 10. Clinical characteristics of the patients affecting distant recurrence in univariate and multivariate analysis (Cox regression model)

Factor		median survival (month)	univariate analysis (p value)	Hazard ratio (95% CI*)	multivariate analysis (p value)	Hazard ratio (95% CI)
Gender	male	NR†	0.419	1.36 (0.64, 2.87)	NA‡	
	female	NR				
Age	≥65 years	NR	0.397	1.46 (0.60, 3.56)	NA	
	<65 years	NR				
Pathology	NSCLC§	NR	0.734	1.14 (0.54, 2.40)	NA	
	non-NSCLC	NR				
Extracranial metastasis	presence	NR	0.083	1.89 (0.91, 3.62)	NA	
	absence	NR				
Status of cancer	under-control	NR	*0.005*	2.61 (1.29, 5.26)	*0.023*	2.89 (1.16, 7.23)
	out-of-control	11.4				
KPS□ score	≥70	NR	*0.034*	2.70 (1.04, 7.03)	0.863	1.20 (0.15, 9.94)
	<70	NR				
Postoperative radiotherapy	yes	NR	0.278	1.55 (0.70, 3.46)	0.383	1.58 (0.57, 4.38)
	no	11.6				

CI*; confidence interval, NR†; not reached at median value, NA‡; not assessed, NSCLC§; non-small cell lung cancer, KPS□; Karnofsky Performance Scale

Table 11. Features of the brain metastasis affecting distant recurrence in univariate and multivariate analysis (Cox regression model)

Factor		median survival (month)	univariate analysis (month)	Hazard ratio (95% CI*)	multivariate analysis (month)	Hazard ratio (95% CI)
Timing of metastasis	synchronous	NR†	0.458	1.30 (0.65, 2.62)	NA‡	
	metachronous	NR				
Tumor size	<3cm	NR	0.570	1.24 (0.59, 2.62)	NA	
	≥3cm	NR				
Tumor locations	supratentorial	NR	0.230	2.04 (0.62, 6.70)	NA	
	infratentorial	NR				
Method of surgery	MCR§	NR	0.071	1.94 (0.93, 4.02)	0.173	1.87 (0.76, 4.59)
	GTR□	11.6				

CI*; confidence interval, NR†; not reached at median value, NA‡; not assessed, MCR§; microscopic complete resection, GTR□; gross total resection

DISCUSSION

In this study, we found that local recurrence can be markedly reduced by the wide resection of BM including microscopic, infiltrative tumor cells surrounding a tumor with confirming clean surgical margin by intraoperative margin biopsy. Metastatic brain tumors are commonly circumscribed, although not actually capsulated, and can often be totally separated from neighboring brain tissue. During surgery, after the location of a lesion has been identified, a cortical incision is preferably made in the depths of the sulcus overlying the tumor. When the gliotic pseudo-capsule of a tumor is reached, the tumor tends to be gradually enucleated from its bed. It is interesting to note, although brain metastasis appears to be well demarcated from surrounding brain tissue on gross examination, that these tumors may have a microscopic infiltrative appearance [5, 21, 22]. In two old autopsy reports, residual tumors were found at the sites of previous surgical excisions in 25% and 42% of cases; moreover, postoperative radiation was not used in these two series [6, 21]. This infiltration is not so extensive as that of malignant gliomas, but nevertheless, it may play an important role in local recurrence after surgical excision.

We have no data on how much surrounding brain should be suctioned out. In brain metastases, however, the tumor invasion distance usually is not >5 mm, as described in the literature. Thus, we decided to resect surrounding brain tissue to at least 5 mm in depth. Actually, we do not have any statistically accurate data on how many frozen sections of the tumor margin were positive for cancer, although up to ~ 10–15% of the biopsy samples were positive for tumor cells. In each case, our pathologists studied 6–10 margin biopsy samples. Additional surgical time needed to perform the pathological analyses would be <30 minutes.

Therefore, we considered that the wide surgical resection of BM including the removal of adjacent tumor cells infiltrating parenchyma and then confirming clean surgical margin during surgery may establish a local cure and diminish local recurrence.

Although many studies have addressed the factors that influence the therapeutic results obtained when BM from lung cancer is treated using different therapeutic modalities, no comprehensive study has assessed the influence of surgical extent on recurrence and survival in patients with BM. The incidence of local recurrence after BM excision in many series is around 40% [23, 24]. However, in the present study, only nine recurrences (19.1%) occurred at a site treated by tumor resection including tumor cells infiltrating adjacent brain parenchyma, even without postoperative brain irradiation. The reason for successful local control in the present study is attributed the absence of a remnant tumor burden due to microscopic complete resection, including microscopic and infiltrative tumor cells adjacent brain parenchyma.

Despite the excellent local control rate achieved in this study, distant CNS relapse rate was as high as 44.7% in the patients who underwent microscopic complete resection, which was similar to other studies [14, 15]. And median survival was only 13.10 months. In terms of survival, reported periods after surgery for BM ranged from 8 to 20 months [4, 10-12, 18, 27]. Moreover, little difference was found between the two groups in this context (median survival time; 13.1 months in group A vs 12.1 months in group B, $p = 0.309$). As expected, patients with a higher performance status at presentation had a longer survival. This study shows that excellent local control of BM, although necessary for prolonged survival, is not sufficient alone to ensure long-term survival. Long-term survival will be achieved only when concurrent advances are made in treatment of local and distant CNS disease and the systemic cancer.

Table 12. Summary of associated factors with survival, local recurrence and distant recurrences

Outcome		univariate analysis	multivariate analysis
Survival	characteristics of patients	gender age KPS* score	gender age KPS score
	features of brain lesions	(-)	(-)
Local recurrence	characteristics of patients	KPS score	(-)
	features of brain lesions	method of surgery	method of surgery
Distant recurrence	characteristics of patients	status of cancer KPS score	status of cancer
	features of brain lesions	(-)	(-)

KPS*; Karnofsky Performance Scale

In the view of this point, Macchiarini et al. showed that systemic chemotherapy was the most significant independent predictor of disease-free long-term survival after neurosurgical resection of BM [9]. These days, many authors consider systemic chemotherapy an important therapeutic modality that offers therapeutic benefit to patients with BM [17, 20, 25, 26]. In the present study, few CNS-related deaths occurred, and most of deaths were attributable to primary cancer progression. Thus, in the context of cause of death in patients with BM, our findings indicate that early and optimal therapy for primary cancer is critically needed.

In fact, the goal of treatment of BM is to eliminate the metastasis and prevent recurrence of tumor in the brain. For patients with BM, despite significant advances in local control, treatment of primary cancer has the most important role in prolonging overall survival [2]. In the present study, the factors influencing survival were not features of brain metastasis, but clinical conditions of patients. Additionally, as our results showed that poorly-controlled primary cancer had higher distant recurrence rate than well-controlled primary tumor, the only factor affecting distant recurrence was status of primary tumor. Therefore, in order to prolong survival and reduce distant recurrence, it is most important to control systemic disease. Thus, one of the most important advantages conferred by microscopic complete resection is that it allows systemic chemotherapy to be started sooner to control both primary cancer and brain metastasis and may establish local cure or complete remission of brain disease.

Class I evidence indicates that brain radiation therapy is the optimal choice for patients with metastatic brain tumors. We also used radiation therapy for the patients with brain metastases. In some cases of NSCLC, however, we initially performed systemic chemotherapy postoperatively for the early control of the primary disease. Brain radiotherapy was delayed until a local brain recurrence developed. In cases of small, deep-seated, surgically inaccessible tumors, uncontrolled primary disease, or a KPS score too poor for general anesthesia, we also performed radiosurgery

Conclusion

The present study provides the first published description of surgical outcome for wide surgical resection of BM including microscopic infiltrative cancer cells adjacent brain parenchyma with confirming clean surgical margin by intraoperative margin biopsy. This study shows that wide surgical resection of BM with confirming clean surgical margin during surgery can reduce local recurrence markedly.

Acknowledgments

The authors thank Young Min Kim, M.D. and Mi-Ok Sunwoo, M.D. (Department of Radiology, Samsung Changwon Hospital) for their review of the neuroradiological images; Mi Hyeon Jin, B.S. (Department of Biostatistics, Samsung Changwon Hospital) for assistance with the statistical analysis; Mee Seon Kim, M.D. (Department of Pathology) for her pathological review; and Tae Gyu Kim, M.D. (Department of Radiation Oncology, Samsung Changwon Hospital) for delivering the radiotherapy detailed in this work.

Disclosure

This study was financially supported by a Samsung Biomedical Research Institute grant (SMX-1151291). The authors report no conflict of interest concerning the materials or methods used in this study or the findings specified in this paper.

REFERENCES

[121] Andreas MS, Hauke T, Ralf B, Janka HF, Maximilian MH (2005). Surgical treatment for brain metastases; Prognostic factors and survival in 177 patients. *Neurosurg Rev* 28, 115-119.

[122] Andrews DW, Scott CB, Sperduto PW, Flanders AE, Gaspar LE, Schell MC, et al. (2004). Whole brain radiation therapy with or without stereotactic radiosurgery boost for patients with one to three brain metastases: Phase III results of the RTOG 9508 randomized trial. Lancet 363, 1665-1672.

[123] Gaspar L, Scott C, Rotman M, Asbell S, Phillips T, Wasserman T, et al. (1997). Recursive partitioning analysis (RPA) of prognostic factors in three Radiation Therapy Oncology Group (RTOG) brain metastases trials. *Int J Radiat Oncol Biol Phys* 37, 745-751.

[124] Hankins JR, Miller JE, Scalcman M, Ferraro F, Green DC, Attar S, et al. (1988). Surgical management of lung cancer with solitary cerebral metastasis. *Ann Thorac Surg* 46, 24-28.

[125] Henson R, Urich H. (Eds.): Cancer and Nervous System. London: Blackwell. 1982.

[126] Lang EF, Slater J (1964). Metastatic brain tumors: Results of surgical and nonsurgical treatment. *Surg Clin North Am* 44, 865.

[127] Lang Frederick F, Chang Eric L, Abis-Said Dima, Wildrick David M, Sawaya Raymond: Metastatic brain tumors in Youmans JR (ed.): Neurological Surgery, ed 5. Philadelphia: WB Saunders, 2003, Vol 1, pp1077-1097.

[128] Larson D, Rubenstein J, McDermott M: Treatment of metastatic cancer, in DeVita VT Jr, Hellman S, Rosenberg SA (eds): Cancer Principles and Practice of Oncology. Philadelphia: Lippincott Williams and Wilkins, 2004, pp 2323-2398.

[129] Macchiarini P, Bronaguidi R, Hardin M, Mussi A, Angeletti CA (1991). Results and prognostic factors of surgery in the management of non-small-cell-lung cancer with brain metastases. *Cancer* 68, 300-304.

[130] Magilligan DJ, Duvernoy C, Malik G, Lewis JW, Knighton R, Ausman JI (1986). Surgical approach to lung cancer with solitary cerebral metastasis; twenty-five years' experience. *Ann Thorac Surg* 42, 360-364.

[131] Matthhew GE, Steven B, Mark G, Robbert G, Paul LP, Mahesh V, et al. (2007). Treatment of single brain metastasis with resection, intracavity carmustine polymer wafers and radiation therapy is safe and provides excellent local control. *Clin Cancer Res* 13(12), 3637-3641.

[132] Mussi A, Pistolesi M, Lucchi M, Janni A, Chella A, Parenti G, et al. (1996). Resection of single brain metastasis in non-small cell lung cancer: prognostic factor. *J Thorac Cardiovasc Surg* 112(1), 146-153.

[133] Paek SH, Audu PB, Sperling MR, Cho J, Andrew DW (2005). Reevaluation of surgery for the treatment of brain metastases; Review of 208 patients with single or multiple brain metastases treated at one institution with modern neurological techniques. *Neurosurgery* 56, 1021-1034.

[134] Patchell RA, Tibbs PA, Regine WF, Dempsey RJ, Mohiuddin M, Kryscio RJ, et al. (1998). Postoperative radiotherapy in the treatment of single metastases to the brain: a randomized trial. *JAMA* 280, 1485-1489.

[135] Patchell RA, Tibbs PA, Walsh JW (1990). A randomized trial of surgery in the treatment of single metastases to the brain. *N Engl J Med* 322, 494-500.

[136] Posner JB, Chernik NL (1978). Intracranial metastases from systemic cancer. *Adv Neurol* 19, 579-592.

[137] Postmus P.E, Smit E.F: Chemotherapy for brain metastases of lung cancer; A review. Ann Oncol 10 : 753-759, 1999.

[138] Salvati M, Cervoni L, Delfini R (1996). Solitary brain metastases from non-oat cell lung cancer: clinical and prognostic factors. *Neurosurg Rev* 19(4), 221-225.

[139] Sawaya R, Hammoud M, Schoppa D, Hess KR, Wu SZ, Shi WM, et al. (1998). Neurosurgical outcomes in a modern series of 400 craniotomies for treatment of parenchymal tumors. *Neurosurgery* 42(5), 1044-1055.

[140] Soffietti R, Costanza A, Laguzzi E, Nobile M, Ruda R (2005). Radiotherapy and chemotherapy of brain metastases. *J Neurooncol* 75 : 31-42.

[141] Stortebecker TP (1954). Metastatic tumors of the brain from a neurosurgical point of view: A follow-up study of 158 cases. *J Neurosurg* 11, 84.

[142] Sundaresan N, Galicich JH (1985). Surgical treatment of brain metastases; Clinical and computerized tomography evaluation of the results of treatment. *Cancer* 55 : 1382-1388.

[143] Sundaresan N, Galicichi JH (1985). Surgical treatment of single brain metastases from non-small cell lung cancer. *Cancer Invest* 3, 207.

[144] Sundaresan N, Sachdev VP, DiGiacinto GV, Hyghes JE (1988). Reoperation for brain metastases. *J Clin Oncol* 6, 1625-1629.
[145] van den Bent M.J (2003). The role of chemotherapy in brain metastases. *Eur J Cancer* 39, 2114-2120.
[146] Wolfgang Schuette (2004). Treatment of brain metastases from lung cancer: Chemotherapy. *Lung Cancer* 45 (Suppl. 2), S253-S257.
[147] Wronsky M, Arbit E, Burt M, Galicich JH (1996). Survival after surgical treatment of brain metastases from lung cancer; a follow-up study of 231 patients treated between 1976 and 1991. *J Neurosurg* 83, 605-616.

Biographical Sketch

Young Zoon Kim, M.D., Ph.D.

Affiliation: Sungkyunkwan University School of Medicine, Samsung Changwon Hospital, Division of Neurooncology and Department of Neurosurgery

Education:

- March 2008-August 2012: Ph.D. in Medicine, Dong-A University, Graduate School of Medicine, Busan, Republic of Korea
- March 2006-February 2008: M.S. in Medicine, Dong-A University, Graduate School of Medicine, Busan, Republic of Korea
- March 1992-February 2000: B.S. in Medicine, Busan National University School of Medicine, Busan, Republic of Korea

Address: 158 Paryong-ro, Masanhoewon-gu, Changwon, 51353, Korea. Sungkyunkwan University School of Medicine, Samsung Changwon Hospital Division of Neurooncology and Department of Neurosurgery

Research and professional experience:

January 2006	2006 Investigator Training Course, Asan Medical Center Clinical Research Center (Basic Course)
February 2006	Advance Course of Training Bioscience Research, National Cancer Center, Korea
January 2007	2007 Investigator Training Course, Asan Medical Center

	Clinical Research Center (Advanced Course)
February 2007	Advance Course of Hospice Manager, National Cancer Center, Korea
October 2010	2010 KoNECT GCP Training for Investigators (INV-CNT-SMC-1002020)
February 2011	4th Clinical Research Design Course (No. CRDC-11-23) Johns Hopkins University and Samsung Medical Center Clinical Research Center
September 2011	2011 GCP Training for Investigators, Samsung Medical Center Clinical Research Center
November 2011	2011 Advance Clinical Research Design Course (No. ACRDC-003) Johns Hopkins University and Samsung Medical Center Clinical Research Center
July 2013	Animal Care and Use in Research and Education Course (#2782614) AALAS Learning Library in MD Anderson Cancer Center
February 2014	Training program for Brain Tumor Research (BTR 14-0023), Brain Tumor Center, The University of Texas MD Anderson Cancer Center
March 2014	Completion of the Collaborative Institutional Training Initiative (CITI) program (K-2014-12626560) Biomedical Research
November 2015	Completion of Advanced Training Course for Scientific Reviewer of IRB (KAIRB 2015-17009)
March 2016	Completion of the Collaborative Institutional Training Initiative (CITI) program (K-2016-19035082) GCP for Clinical Trials with Drugs and Biologics (K-2016-18171355) Biomedical Research

Professional appointments:

March 2014 ~ present	**Associate Professor**, Department of Neurosurgery, Samsung Changwon Hospital, Samsung Medical Center, Sungkyunkwan University School of Medicine, Changwon, Republic of Korea
March 2009 ~ present	**Director,** Division of Neurooncology, Samsung Changwon Hospital, Samsung Medical Center, Sungkyunkwan University School of Medicine,

	Changwon, Republic of Korea
March 2013 ~ February 2014	**Exchange Professor**, Center for Cancer Epigenetics Department of Molecular Cellular Oncology, MD Anderson Cancer Center, The University of Texas, Houston, TX, USA
March 2009 ~ February 2014	**Assistant Professor**, Department of Neurosurgery, Samsung Changwon Hospital, Samsung Medical Center, Sungkyunkwan University School of Medicine, Changwon, Republic of Korea
March 2007 ~ February 2009	**Faculty Instructor**, Department of Neurosurgery, Samsung Changwon Hospital, Samsung Medical Center, Sungkyunkwan University School of Medicine, Changwon, Republic of Korea
March 2005 ~ February 2007	**Fellow,** Department of Neurooncology, National Cancer Center Hospital and Research Institute, Goyang, Republic of Korea
March 2001 ~ February 2005	**Resident,** Department of Neurosurgery, Dong-A University Medical Center, Busan, Republic of Korea
March 2000 ~ February 2001	**Medical Intern**, Dong-A University Medical Center, Busan, Republic of Korea

Honors:

March 2010	Best Investigator Award by In-Sung Medical Science Research Foundation
July 2010	Travel Award for ACOS by Korean Cancer Association
March 2011	Best Investigator Award by Genomic Research Center (GRC) of Samsung Medical Research Foundation
April 2011	Best Investigator Award by Handok Medical Research Foundation
May 2011	Best Investigator Award by Daewoong Medical Research Foundation
November 2011	Best Investigator Award by Sanofi-Aventis Medical Research Foundation
January 2012	Designation in "Marquis Who's Who in the World, 2012" Best investigator Award by Samsung Biomedical Research Institute (SBRI)
April 2012	"***2000 Outstanding Intellectuals of the 21st Century, 2012***" by International Biographical Center

May 2012	Designation in "***Great Minds of the 21st Century, 6th Edition, 2012***" by American Biographical Institute
June 2012	"***2012 Cancer Academy Award***" by Korean Cancer Association
July 2012	Travel award for EACR 2012 Meeting by Korean Association for Clinical Oncology
November 2012	Travel award for SNO 2012 Meeting by Korean Society for Neuro-Oncology
November 2012	"***Medical Science Award of Excellence 2012***" by American Biographical Institute
January 2013	Designation in "Marquis Who's Who in the World, 2013"
January 2014	Designation in "Great Minds of the 21st Century, 7th Edition, 2013" by American Biographical Institute
June 2014	Designation in "Marquis Who's Who in the World, 2014"
September 2014	Best Investigator Award by Hanmi Medical Research Foundation
	Designation in "Great Minds of the 21st Century, 8th Edition, 2014" by American Biographical Institute
January 2015	Travel award for ASNO 2014 Meeting by Korean Brain Tumor Society
February 2015	Designation in "Marquis Who's Who in the World, 2015"
April 2015	2014 Best Investigator Faculty Award (by President of Sungkyunkwan University)
	Dr. Song Jin-Eon's Memorial Academic Award by Korean Neurosurgical Society (The Best Investigator's Award of Korean Neurosurgical Society)
May 2015	The Creative Research Project Award by Samsung Biomedical Research Institute (SBRI)
November 2015	Travel award for 2015 SNO Meeting by Korean Society for Neuro-Oncology

Publications last 3 years:

1. Kim J, Lee SH, Jang JH, Kim MS, Lee EH, Kim YZ. Overexpression of MLL4 (histone H3 lysine 4 methyltransferase) and UTX (histone H3 lysine 27 demethylase) prolongs the overall survival of glioblastoma patients with methylated MGMT promoter. J Neurosurg [accepted]
2. Kim YZ, Jang JH, Lee EH, Kim KH, Kim CH. The role of cell-cycle regulators on predicting the progression of silent pituitary adenoma after surgical resection. J Neurooncol [2nd revision]

3. Lee YM, Kim YZ. Clinical and radiological benefit of hybrid fixation compared with short segment fixation for the unstable thoracolumbar junction fracture. Revista Kasmera. 44(3): in press, 2016
4. Kim J, Kim YZ. High dose methotrexate-based vincristine and procarbazine combination chemotherapy as front-line treatment for primary CNS lymphoma patients gives a good clinical outcome even without radiotherapy. Revista Kasmera. 44(1): 76-117, 2016
5. Dhar S, Lee SH, Chen K, Zhu G, Oh WK, Allton K, Gafni O, Kim YZ, Barton M, Hanna JH, Wang Z, Li W, Lee MG. An essential role for UTX in resolution and activation of bivalent promoters. Nucleic Acids Res. 2016 Jan 13. pii: gkv1516. [Epub ahead of print]
6. DC Kim, KU Kim, YZ Kim. Prognostic role of methylation status of the MGMT promoter determined quantitatively by pyrosequencing in glioblastoma patients. J Korean Neurosurg Soc 59(1): 26-36, 2016
7. YZ Kim. Protein Methylation and Demethylation in Cancer. Int J Neurol Res 1(3): 79-91, 2015
8. SH Lee, JH Jang, KH Kim, YZ Kim. Stent-assisted Coil Embolization of Petrous Internal Carotid Artery in a Teenager with Neurofibromatosis. J Cerebrovasc Endovasc Neurosurg 17(3): 252-256, 2015
9. SH Lee, EH Lee, SH Lee, YM Lee, HD Kim, YZ Kim. Epigenetic role of histone 3 lysine methyltransferase and demethylase in regulating apoptosis predicting the recurrence of atypical meningioma. J Korean Med Sci 30(8):1157-1166, 2015
10. YZ Kim, JH Kwon, S Lim. A clinical analysis of brain metastasis in gynecologic cancer: A retrospective multi-institute analysis. J Kor Med Sci 30(1): 66-73, 2015
11. MS Kim, KH Kim, EH Lee, YM Lee, SH Lee, HD Kim, YZ Kim. Results of immunohistochemical staining for cell cycle regulators predict the recurrence of atypical meningiomas. J Neurosurg 121: 1189-1200, 2014
12. MS Kim, YM Lee, JS Kim, YZ Kim. Erosive perforation of bladder with calculus formation as a complication of ventriculo-peritoneal shunt. J Kor Soc Geriat Neurosurg 10 (1): 54-57, 2014
13. YZ Kim. Altered histone modifications in gliomas. Brain Tumor Res Treat 2(1): 7-21, 2014
14. EH Lee, KH Kim, JH Kwon, HD Kim, YZ Kim. Results of immunohistochemical staining of cell cycle regulators - the prediction of recurrence of functioning pituitary adenoma. World Neurosurg 81(3-4): 563-575, 2014

15. KR Kim, YZ Kim. Clinical comparison of 30-day mortalities and 6-month functional recoveries after spontaneous intracerebral hemorrhage in patients with or without end-stage renal disease. J Korean Neurosurg Soc 54(3): 164-174, 2013
16. KR Kim, YM Lee, YZ Kim, YW Cho, JS Kim, KH Kim, IC Lee. Cervical myelopathy secondary to atlanto-occipital assimilation: The usefulness of the simple decompressive surgery. Korean J Spine 10(3): 189-91, 2013
17. YZ Kim, YH Park, YG Song, KH Kim. Clinical analysis of factors predisposing the recurrence of primary intracerebral hemorrhage in patients taking anti-hypertensive drugs: A prospective cohort study. Clin Neurol Neurosurg 115(5): 578-586, 2013
18. KH Kim, HD Kim, YZ Kim. Comparisons of 30-day mortalities and 90-day functional recoveries after first and recurrent primary intracerebral hemorrhage attacks: A multi-institute based retrospective study. World Neurosurg 79(3-4): 489-498, 2013

In: Horizons in Cancer Research. Volume 63 ISBN: 978-1-53610-013-6
Editor: Hiroto S. Watanabe

Chapter 3

TRENDS OF COMPUTER-AIDED DIAGNOSIS IN ESTIMATING TUMOR MALIGNANCY

Chung-Ming Lo[1,*] and Ng Kee Koon[2]
[1]Graduate Institute of Biomedical Informatics, College of Medical Science and Technology, Taipei Medical University, Taipei, Taiwan
[2]Graduate Institute of Clinical Medicine,
Taipei Medical University, Taipei, Taiwan

ABSTRACT

This chapter encapsulates the trends of the computer-aided diagnosis (CAD) development for the estimation of tumor malignancy. Due to the high occurrence rate of cancer, more and more abnormal cell growth can appear at any organs in human body. To avoid unnecessary biopsy, the malignancy evaluation should be modeled and acquired via noninvasive examinations. CADs based on medical images are the effective tool for this purpose. Upon the developments of imaging modalities, more and more tumor characteristics can be observed and quantified. As an adjunct to mammography in breast cancer. Ultrasound techniques including B-mode, Doppler, elastogaphy are proposed to extract the physical, mechanical properties, and vessel distribution around tumors. Based on the artificial intelligence classifier, the complementary power of various features can be combined to deal with the heterogeneity of cancer types. These quantitative features can be classified into two categories:

* Corresponding author: buddylo@tmu.edu.tw.

morphology and texture features. For ultrasound images, the echogenicities of different tissues are presented by gray-scale pixel values. The gray-scale intensities of region of interest can be analyzed without image segmentation or manual delineation and thus especially convenient for texture analysis. However, different settings or manufactures of ultrasound scanners usually result in different gray-scale distributions for the same tissue. The newly developed intensity-invariant texture features based on multi-resolution and orientations which successfully classified breast tumors into benign and malignant groups with accuracy higher than 80% are introduced as a solution. Finally, the use of CAD can be extended to precision medicine. Gene expression of everyone is quite different due to the inherent and environmental effects. In the past, the researches about gene are isolated to clinical examinations because the cost and the invasive procedures. With the development of image features extracted from medical images such as computed tomography, magnetic resonance imaging, ultrasound, and so on, the correlations between hundreds of quantitative image features and gene expressions are explored. The success of the researches can discover more tumor characteristics from image properties to gene expression for cancer stage estimation, survival rate, and many related issues. The role of CAD would be more important than before because of the computation of more data and more sophisticated techniques.

1. Introduction

Cancers are asymptomatic at early stages. The initial presentation, screening method and diagnosis depends on cancer type and location. In the case of breast cancer, the exterior location makes it possible for early detection of lump by palpation. Medical images based on X-ray, ultrasound or MRI is attained to support clinical diagnosis for visualization of tumor shape, margin, orientation, and composition. In addition to medical history such as tumor growth rate, tumor shape, presence of skin or nipple retraction, and painless axillary lymphadenopathy, physician often relies heavily on medical image to decide whether to attain a biopsy proof.

Medical image is a reliable tool for early cancer detection. Breast cancer is the second most common cancer-related cause of death for adult [1]. Early detection of breast cancer not only improves the prognosis of patients [2], but also reduces health care spending. Since human fingertips are only sensitive to larger lump size of 0.5cm and above, a better tool such as mammography with a higher sensitivity on detection of smaller mass is a more efficient way of early breast cancer screening in high-risk group. In the last three to four decades, breast cancer death was reduced as a result of mammography screening in high-risk group [3-7]. Due to the concern of radiation exposure and difficulty in mammography result interpretation on dense breast, bilateral screening ultrasound was introduced and shown to be a feasible screening tool with promising result [8-12]. As early screening were shown to be effective, huge amount of medical images were generated. There was relentless effort to develop automated computer-aided diagnosis (CAD) system acted as second reader for these medical images.

CAD system as second helper to radiologists was proposed to reduce oversight error and increase diagnostic accuracy. The values of CAD system in cancer diagnosis lie in accuracy, reproducibility and relief of operator-dependency. In previous studies, CAD system relieved the clinical demand and improved clinician's performance for breast tumor histological classification [13, 14]. The Breast Imaging Reporting and Data System (BI-RADS) lexicon was developed by American College of Radiology since 2003 to standardize the terminology and description of breast tumor. There were attempts to extract BI-RADS lexicon features including shape, orientation, margin, lesion boundary, echo pattern, and posterior acoustic characteristics to differentiate benign and malignant tumor [15]. In the first section, strain features of elastography were added into the CAD system composed of B-mode image features such as shape, size, orientation, and echogenic texture based on GLCM [16]. The quantified properties of tissue stiffness are considered in a CAD system because tissue stiffness is intuitively an important part of clinical examination on breast tumor. It is demonstrated that the addition of dimensions to data improves precision and accuracy of disease detection. In the second section, a CAD system was developed for classification of benign and malignant for BI-RADS category 3 [17]. When the features assimilating BI-RADS lexicon was first used, the effectiveness of texture analysis seemed to be falling behind [17]. Unlike other features such as shape, size, and orientation; texture features extraction often requires further pre-processing. Methodologies of texture analysis based on intensity-invariant approach and speckles feature extraction are shown with automated segmentation [18]. Masotti's ranklet transform is the basis of this intensity-invariant approach. Rank is first assigned to each pixel or voxel based on intensity. Then, texture features were extracted by Haralick's gray-level co-occurrence matrix (GLCM) [19]. Multi-resolution and orientation-selective is achieved with invariant to gray-scale variations [20]. This approach was initially used on mammography and found to reduce false-positive rate significantly [19]. Due to system independence of intensity-invariant approach, it is a suitable texture analysis approach of ultrasonography. In the third section, features were extracted from MRI images of malignant breast tumor and correlated with genomic data including copy number variations, somatic mutation, protein expression, miRNA expression and transcriptional activities [21]. The quantified phenotypes of tumor include size, shape, margin, and blood flow kinetics. Large-scale comparison and correlation of molecular pathway and medical image acquired tumor phenotypes in breast cancer was demonstrated for the first time. This created not only a way to understand tumor biology, but also to bridge and extend the role of CAD system into tumor biology based diagnostic and prognosis monitoring tool.

Malignant tumor is composed of heterogeneous cell types dynamically affected by treatment. Medical images feature including shape, size, and heterogeneity have been used as a mean to observe extend of tumor response to treatment. Compared with laboratory test, genomic and proteomic assays; quantified image features provide unique set of information on tumor phenotype and microenvironment reflecting the underlying pathophysiology. The practice of medical image conversion into quantitative features is called radiomics. Instead of using standard-of-care image for visual interpretation, features from volume of interest are extracted for medical decision support. In the pursuit of precision medicine, radiomics offers a unique tool to study tumor biology in clinical setting noninvasively and longitudinally. The feasibility of radiomics was tested and promising result was shown in distinguishing prostate cancer from benign prostate tissue [22], characterization of glioblastoma multiforme [23], clear cell renal cell carcinoma [24], lung and head-and-neck cancer [25]. Although radiomics is still in early stage of development and the robustness of features are still in the process of testing, it fills in the gap of tumor biology study and potentially acted as an approach to perfect clinical diagnosis.

2. The Integration of Qualitatiave BI-RADS and Quantitative Strain Features in Elastography

2.1. Introduction of Elastography

Elastography record tissue stiffness through application of stress (σ) and measurement of tissue deformation (or strain, ε). Elasticity is mathematically expressed as Young's modulus, $E = \sigma/\varepsilon$. The stress could be applied by operator or passively through patient's respirator movement to minimize operator-dependency. The elastography image acquired in this study is composed of 8-bit gray-scale image with softness close to 255 (white color), and hardness close to 0 (black color).

2.2. Data Acquisition

This retrospective study involved 90 patients with half benign and the other half malignant core needle biopsy-proven cases. Detailed information of tumor histology, lesion size and patient age are included in Table 1. The B-mode and elastography images were attainted by Ultrasonography model ACUSON S2000 (Siemens Medical Solutions, Mountain View, CA) with 9L4 linear-array transducer. The acquisition of elastography is based on eSie Touch technique where deformation is induced by patient's respiratory movement with probe lightly place in contact with skin. Both B-mode and elastography images are 8-bit gray-scale image.

Table 1. Detailed information of cases

	Malignant		Benign	
Sample size	45		45	
Age	39-83 (54 ± 12 years old)		18-80 (44 ± 12 years old)	
Lesion size	1.37 ± 0.39cm		1.21 ± 0.73cm	
Histology	Invasive ductal carcinoma	37	Fibroadenoma	23
	Invasive lobular carcinoma	2	Fibrocystic change	14
	Ductal carcinoma *in situ*	6	Intraductal Papilloma	8

2.3. Tumor Segmentation

The original B-mode and elastography images are shown in Figure 1. Sigmoid filter [26] is first applied to original B-mode image to strengthen the tumor edge. After the processed image is passed through gradient magnitude filter [27], sigmoid filtering is performed again for suppression of speckle noise while conserving tumor contour that possessed strong intensity gap. Tumor contour is acquired by level-set segmentation method [28] which is a semi-automatic method that require user-defined seed in tumor area. Through propagation from this user-defined seed, tumor contour is delineated and mapped on the elastography image.

2.4. Strain Features

The delineated tumor contour in B-mode image is mapped on elastography image. The following two strain features are extracted in this delineated region.

$$\text{StrainMean} = \left(\sum_{E(i,j)\in T} E(GrayScale)\right)/TN \quad (1)$$

$$\text{StrainVar} = \frac{StrainMean}{\left(\sum_{E(i,j)\in T} \; (E(GrayScale)-StrainMean)^2\right)/TN} \quad (2)$$

Where *StrainMean* [29, 30] is the average gray-scale values E(i, j) from original elastography within tumor contour. The summation of gray-scale values in tumor contour (T) is divided by total number of pixels (TN). This feature represents the average stiffness within tumor area. *StrainVAR* [29-32] measures the variance of stiffness within tumor region. A higher variation of stiffness in the tumor contour resulted in smaller value of *StrainVAR*. This is an effective term to describe stiffness heterogeneity in within tumor. The alternation of tumor stiffness associates with angiogenesis and necrosis, both are the histological signs of malignancy [33].

The difference in tumor area in B-mode and stiff strain region in elastography has long been used for distinguishing malignant and benign [29, 34-37]. Malignancy is likely suggested when the strain-to-B-mode ratio greater than 1.0. The alternation of stiffness in peri-tumor area is associated with desmoplastic reaction of stromal cell and abundant collagens

y and variance of normalized radial length (NRL entropy and variance). Normalized Radial Length (NRL) is based on ean distance from the center of the tumor to margin [48].
er of speculation on tumor contour (SpiculationNum)
ty difference around tumor boundary (LB), between tumor and nding tissue (EP_Outer) and posterior area (PS)
enic texture of GLCM includes Energy, Correlation, Cluster , Cluster Prominence and Haralick Correlation; standard ion and average (as discussed in section 3.5).

and Discussion

e 6 strain features and 16 B-mode extracted features. The f each features were assessed by Kolmogorov-Smirnov test. n the distribution, Student's t-test or Mann-Whitney U-test was selection of statistically significant (p-value < 0.05) features on c regression model. Most of the strain features were statistically in differentiating malignant and benign tumor, except *Level*. All 16 B-mode extracted features were statistically tumor characterization.

ic model was constructed by binary logistic regression model features, B-mode features, or both. Feature selection was ith backward stepwise elimination. Features that produce minimal sidual error sum of squares were removed. Leave-one-out cross-nethod was performed on the selected features to examine the ower. Comparing the prediction result with biopsy-proven result, 5 indices including accuracy, sensitivity, specificity, positive alue (PPV), negative predictive value (NPV); were calculated and Table 2. Chi-Square was utilized for evaluation of statistical . The result in Table 2 indicates strain features out-performed B-ures. The additional of strain features with B-mode features y improved Az from 0.70 to 0.93.

accumulation. Desmoplastic reaction is extracellular matrix remodeling process of stromal cell. It is generally perceived as the initiation of cancer invasion and metastasis. Strain-to-B-mode difference is important for tumor characterization and commonly practiced by radiologist [29, 34-39]. Visual scoring system was developed based on this concept [40]. As it is the case in most visual scoring system, great interobserver variability was demonstrated [34]. With the assistance of programming, this important feature can be quantified according to B-mode and elastography image. Other important strain-to-B-mode features include stiffness contrast and normalized shear strain area [29, 38, 39, 41-43]. Stiffness contrast represents the ratio of strain mean within masses and background. Normalized shear strain is the strain mean within tumor normalized with tumor size.

The size ratio between B-mode tumor area and FCM-cluster strain image area is expression in the following equation

$$LengthRatio = \frac{length(j_{\max}, B_{FCM})}{length(j_{\max}, T_{B\,mode})}, j_{\max} = \arg\max \; length(j, T_{B\,mode}) \quad (3)$$

j_{max} is the row with maximum tumor length in delineated tumor region of B-mode ($T_{B\,mode}$). The length of such term is the denominator. FCM clustering is first performed in elastography image. The length of FCM clustered black region in elastography image is corresponded to j_{max}, forming the numerator term (the red line in Figure 2).

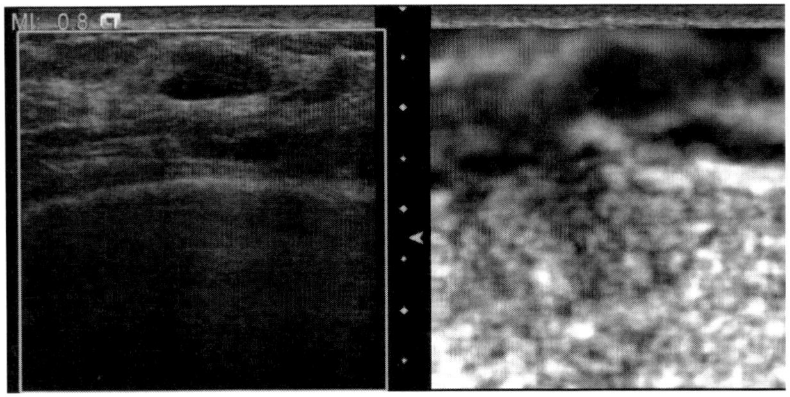

Figure 1. Original B-mode (left) and Elastography (right) image.

GlobalDarkLevel and *GlobalStrainLevel* are second-order statistical strain features along the upper and lower boundary of tumor contour delineated in B-mode image. *GlobalDarkLevel* is the total number of black pixel in FCM-clustered elastography image enclosed by the upper and lower bound of tumor contour. *GlobalStrainLevel* is the summation of all gray-scale pixel values in the same region.

$$\text{GlobalDarkLevel} = \sum B_{FCM}(i,j), j \geq argmin\, row(T_{Bmode}), j \leq argmax\, row(T_{Bmode}) \quad (4)$$

$$\text{GlobalDarkLevel} = \sum E(i,j), j \geq argmin\, row(T_{Bmode}), j \leq argmax\, row(T_{Bmode}) \quad (5)$$

2.5. Fuzzy C-Means (FCM) Clustering of Strain Features

FCM clustering [28, 44] was applied to categorization of 8-bit gray-scale elastography image into 0, 128, and 255 represented by black, gray, and white color in Figure 2. FCM clustering assigns each pixel based on gray-scale intensity and equalization of pixel count in each cluster. The following function is minimized to achieve such classification:

$$\text{J} = \sum_{i=1}^{N} \sum_{j=1}^{C} u_{ij}^{m} \left\| x_i - c_j \right\|^2 \quad (6)$$

Where N is the total number of pixel in the image. C is the total number of clusters. In this case, C = 3. x_i is the gray-scale value of individual pixel. c_j is a temporary gray-scale value of centroid pixel of cluster j. The centroid value of c_j is refined each iteration by Equation 22. u_{ij} is the membership of gray-scale value difference between x_i and c_j. In Equation 23, u_{ij} characterizes how close x_i is to centroid of cluster c_j over centroid c_j where j and k are not equal. m is an under-defined variable. FCM clustering algorithm is initiated by the summation of u_{ij} membership of x_i to c_j of each cluster is equal to 1 [45-47]:

$$\sum_{j=1}^{c} u_{ij} = 1, \forall j = 1 \ldots c \quad (7)$$

$$c_j = \frac{\sum_{i=1}^{N} u_{ij}^{m} \cdot x_i}{\sum_{i=1}^{N} u_{ij}^{m}} \quad (8)$$

$$u_{ij} = -$$

The iterations stop when J of Eq
chosen in each clusters resulted in
minimum sum of difference between

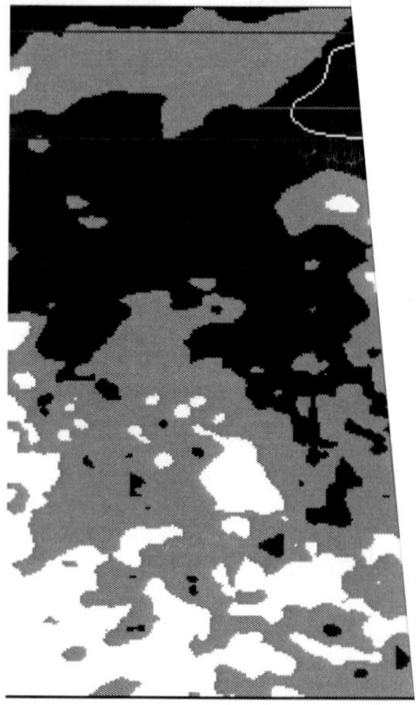

Figure 2. Fuzzy c-means (FCM) clustering of el
Tumor contour segmented from B-mode image
illustrates the maximum diameter of tumor regic
the strain area defined by delineated tumor widtl

2.6. B-mode Features

The extracted B-mode features in this stu

1. Tumor area in delineated tumor conto
2. Minor axis length (Ellipse_b) and th best-fit eclipse (Ellipse_compact)

3. Entrop NRL Euclid
4. Numb
5. Intens surrou
6. Echog Shade deviat

2.7. Results

There ar distribution c Depending o used for pre- binary logisti significant *GlobalStrain* significant in

Diagnos with strain performed w predictive re validation n prediction p performanc predictive v shown in significanc mode feat significantl

accumulation. Desmoplastic reaction is extracellular matrix remodeling process of stromal cell. It is generally perceived as the initiation of cancer invasion and metastasis. Strain-to-B-mode difference is important for tumor characterization and commonly practiced by radiologist [29, 34-39]. Visual scoring system was developed based on this concept [40]. As it is the case in most visual scoring system, great interobserver variability was demonstrated [34]. With the assistance of programming, this important feature can be quantified according to B-mode and elastography image. Other important strain-to-B-mode features include stiffness contrast and normalized shear strain area [29, 38, 39, 41-43]. Stiffness contrast represents the ratio of strain mean within masses and background. Normalized shear strain is the strain mean within tumor normalized with tumor size.

The size ratio between B-mode tumor area and FCM-cluster strain image area is expression in the following equation

$$LengthRatio = \frac{length(j_{\max}, B_{FCM})}{length(j_{\max}, T_{B\,mode})}, j_{\max} = \arg\max\ length(j, T_{B\,mode}) \tag{3}$$

j_{max} is the row with maximum tumor length in delineated tumor region of B-mode ($T_{B\,mode}$). The length of such term is the denominator. FCM clustering is first performed in elastography image. The length of FCM clustered black region in elastography image is corresponded to j_{max}, forming the numerator term (the red line in Figure 2).

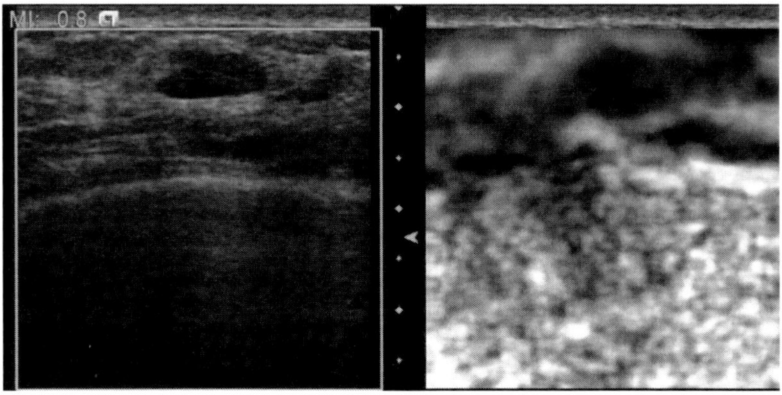

Figure 1. Original B-mode (left) and Elastography (right) image.

GlobalDarkLevel and *GlobalStrainLevel* are second-order statistical strain features along the upper and lower boundary of tumor contour delineated in B-mode image. *GlobalDarkLevel* is the total number of black pixel in FCM-clustered elastography image enclosed by the upper and lower bound of tumor contour. *GlobalStrainLevel* is the summation of all gray-scale pixel values in the same region.

$$\text{GlobalDarkLevel} = \sum^{B_{FCM}(i,j), j \geq argmin\, row(T_{Bmode}), \; j \leq argmax\, row(T_{Bmode})} \quad (4)$$

$$\text{GlobalDarkLevel} = \sum^{E(i,j), j \geq argmin\, row(T_{Bmode}), \; j \leq argmax\, row(T_{Bmode})} \quad (5)$$

2.5. Fuzzy C-Means (FCM) Clustering of Strain Features

FCM clustering [28, 44] was applied to categorization of 8-bit gray-scale elastography image into 0, 128, and 255 represented by black, gray, and white color in Figure 2. FCM clustering assigns each pixel based on gray-scale intensity and equalization of pixel count in each cluster. The following function is minimized to achieve such classification:

$$J = \sum_{i=1}^{N} \sum_{j=1}^{C} u_{ij}^{m} \left\| x_i - c_j \right\|^2 \quad (6)$$

Where N is the total number of pixel in the image. C is the total number of clusters. In this case, C = 3. x_i is the gray-scale value of individual pixel. c_j is a temporary gray-scale value of centroid pixel of cluster *j*. The centroid value of c_j is refined each iteration by Equation 22. u_{ij} is the membership of gray-scale value difference between x_i and c_j. In Equation 23, u_{ij} characterizes how close x_i is to centroid of cluster c_j over centroid c_j where j and k are not equal. *m* is an under-defined variable. FCM clustering algorithm is initiated by the summation of u_{ij} membership of x_i to c_j of each cluster is equal to 1 [45-47]:

$$\sum_{j=1}^{c} u_{ij} = 1, \forall j = 1 \ldots c \quad (7)$$

$$c_j = \frac{\sum_{i=1}^{N} u_{ij}^{m} \cdot x_i}{\sum_{i=1}^{N} u_{ij}^{m}} \quad (8)$$

$$u_{ij} = \frac{1}{\sum_{k=1}^{c}\left(\frac{\|x_i - c_j\|}{\|x_i - c_k\|}\right)^{\frac{2}{m-1}}} \tag{9}$$

The iterations stop when J of Equation 20 is minimized where the centroid chosen in each clusters resulted in almost equal number of pixels. Hence, a minimum sum of difference between pixel values x_i to c_j.

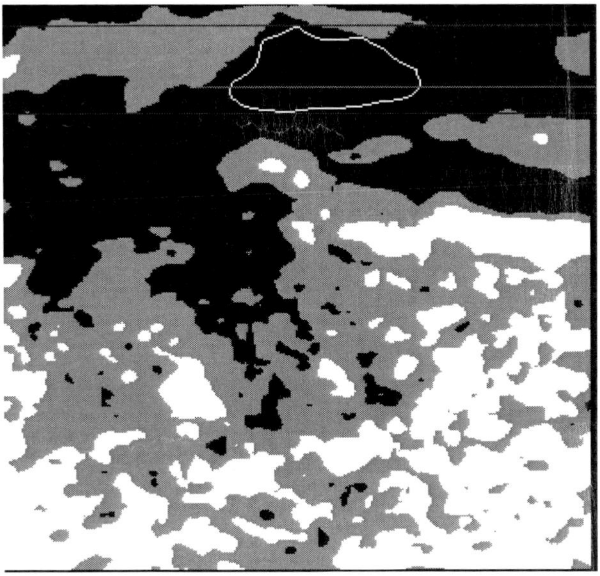

Figure 2. Fuzzy c-means (FCM) clustering of elastography image from Figure 1. Tumor contour segmented from B-mode image is delineated in white line. Red line illustrates the maximum diameter of tumor region in strain image. Blue lines highlight the strain area defined by delineated tumor width.

2.6. B-mode Features

The extracted B-mode features in this study include

1. Tumor area in delineated tumor contour (Tumor_a)
2. Minor axis length (Ellipse_b) and the ratio of perimeter and area in best-fit eclipse (Ellipse_compact)

3. Entropy and variance of normalized radial length (NRL entropy and NRL variance). Normalized Radial Length (NRL) is based on Euclidean distance from the center of the tumor to margin [48].
4. Number of speculation on tumor contour (SpiculationNum)
5. Intensity difference around tumor boundary (LB), between tumor and surrounding tissue (EP_Outer) and posterior area (PS)
6. Echogenic texture of GLCM includes Energy, Correlation, Cluster Shade, Cluster Prominence and Haralick Correlation; standard deviation and average (as discussed in section 3.5).

2.7. Results and Discussion

There are 6 strain features and 16 B-mode extracted features. The distribution of each features were assessed by Kolmogorov-Smirnov test. Depending on the distribution, Student's t-test or Mann-Whitney U-test was used for pre-selection of statistically significant (p-value < 0.05) features on binary logistic regression model. Most of the strain features were statistically significant in differentiating malignant and benign tumor, except *GlobalStrainLevel.* All 16 B-mode extracted features were statistically significant in tumor characterization.

Diagnostic model was constructed by binary logistic regression model with strain features, B-mode features, or both. Feature selection was performed with backward stepwise elimination. Features that produce minimal predictive residual error sum of squares were removed. Leave-one-out cross-validation method was performed on the selected features to examine the prediction power. Comparing the prediction result with biopsy-proven result, 5 performance indices including accuracy, sensitivity, specificity, positive predictive value (PPV), negative predictive value (NPV); were calculated and shown in Table 2. Chi-Square was utilized for evaluation of statistical significance. The result in Table 2 indicates strain features out-performed B-mode features. The additional of strain features with B-mode features significantly improved Az from 0.70 to 0.93.

3. INTENSITY-INVARIANT B-MODE TEXTURE ANALYSIS

3.1. Data Acquisition

This retrospective study involved 69 cases of breast ultrasound BI-RADS category class 3. There were 21 biopsy proven malignant cases and 48 benign cases. A more detailed tumor information including lesion size, histology types are shown in Table 3. The ultrasound images were attained from ATL HDI 3000 (Phillips, Bothell, WA, USA) or Medison Voluson 530 scanner (Kretz Technik, Zipf, Austra). The contrast and brightness setting were not fixed.

Table 2. Assessment of strain features and B-mode extracted features by Chi-Square test

	Performance			p-value		
	Strain	**B-mode**	**Combined**	**Strain vs B-mode**	**Combined vs Strain**	**Combined vs B-mode**
Accuracy	80% (72/90)	68% (61/90)	86% (77/90)	0.0620	0.3236	0.0048*
Sensitivity	80% (36/45)	67% (30/45)	87% (39/45)	0.1527	0.3961	0.0249
Specificity	80% (36/45)	69% (31/45)	84% (38/45)	0.2269	0.5814	0.0811
PPV	80% (36/45)	68% (30/44)	85% (39/46)	0.2029	0.5490	0.0627
NPV	80% (36/45)	67% (31/46)	86% (38/44)	0.1724	0.4227	0.0334
Az	0.84	0.70	0.93	0.0443*	0.0176*	0.0000*

PPV: positive predictive value NPV: negative predictive value
Az: Area under ROC curve * p-value < 0.05

Table 3. Detailed tumor information

	Malignant		Benign	
Sample size	21		48	
Age	28 – 84 (mean = 47.2)		20 – 53 (mean = 39.9)	
Lesion size	1.2 – 4.7 cm (mean = 4.7 cm)		1.4 – 4.3 cm (mean = 2.6cm)	
Histology	Invasive ductal carcinoma		Fibroadenoma	34
	Grade 2	6	Fibrocystic change	13
	Grade 3	15	Papilloma	1

3.2. Automated Tumor Segmentation

Prior to tumor delineation, sigmoid filter was applied to enhance image contrast and strengthen tumor weak edges [26]. After the image is processed by gradient magnitude filter, level-set segmentation was utilized to acquired tumor contour [17].

3.3. Speckle Detection

When ultrasound passes through breast tissue, the ducts and glands scatters the signal and created heterogeneous granular appearing speckles patterns [49]. Speckle in B-mode images were recently proposed as a feature similarly important to morphology features in breast tumor classification [50, 51].

In order to optimize the speckles features, the gray-scale B-mode image of tumor is first converts to exponential distribution with mean-to-standard deviation ratio of 1.0 with the following formula:

$$I(x, y) = 10^{B(x,y)/B_0} \tag{10}$$

Where $I(x, y)$ represents intensity with exponential distribution. $B(x, y)$ is B-mode pixel gray-scale value. B_0 correspond to transducer frequency [52].

Speckle features are detected by a moving 5-by-5 window in intensity image generated by $I(x, y)$ when the intensity exited the mean-to-standard deviation (W_{mSD}) range of 0.8 – 1.2.

$$W_{mean}(x,y) = \sum_{i=-a}^{a}\sum_{j=-a}^{a} I(x+i,y+j) \Big/ (2a+1)^2 \tag{11}$$

$$W_{mSD}(x,y) = \frac{W_{mean}(x,y)}{\sqrt{\sum_{i=-a}^{a}\sum_{j=-a}^{a}(I(x+i,y+j)-W_{mean}(x,y))^2}} \tag{12}$$

For a 5-by-5 window, a equals to 2. W_{mean} represents the average of intensity in this 5-by-5 window. W_{mSD} represents the mean-to-standard deviation value of each pixel in the 5-by-5 windows.

After speckle features detection, ranklet transform is performed. Speckle features are extracted by Haralick's GLCM.

3.4. Ranklet Transforms

Intra-tumor heterogeneity is highly related to tumor aggressiveness, hence, the prognosis of cancer patient [33]. The texture analysis of tumor has long been applied to characterization of tumor [51, 53]. But, different ultrasonography system, probe, and setting imposes changes that are not due to underlying tumor biology. In order to solve this issue, ranklet transform was performed prior to texture feature extraction in mammography [20] and ultrasonography [54]. Instead of extracting features under gray-scale values, each pixel or voxel is ranked according to strength of gray-scale intensity. Figure 3 shows the consistency of texture on ranklet-transformed image R4V, R4H, and R4D when undergoing contrast enchantment, gamma-correction, and histogram equalization while the texture and morphology of tumor changes in gray-scale ultrasound image.

Ranklet transform is performed in the following steps. Firstly, the image is cropped by different resolution. For example, in the case of 8-by-8 image, a resolution of 2, 4, and 8 generates 49, 25 crops, and 1 crop. Each crop equally contains C pixels. Secondly, rank is assigned to each pixel according to gray-scale intensity in the crop. Thirdly, the crop is geometrically split into two subsets vertically, horizontally, or diagonally. In the case of Figure 3, R4V, R4H, and R4D was resolution of 4 and with vertical, horizontal, and diagonal crop. Fourthly, the difference of relative intensity order (*Ro*) in each subset of each crop is calculated by equation (4). $\pi(p)$ is the rank of pixel p. $C/2 \times C/2 = C^2/4$ calculation are made in each crop. Where C is the number pixels in each crop.

$$R_O = \frac{\sum_{p \in Y_O} \pi(p) - {}^{C}/_{4}\left({}^{C}/_{2}+1\right)}{{}^{C^2}/_{8}} - 1, O = V, H, D \tag{13}$$

3.5. Gray-Level Co-Occurrence Matrix (GLCM)

After Ranklet transform, texture features are extracted according to Haralick's GLCM [19]. The proposed texture features are listed in the following: Energy and Local homogeneity measures image homogeneity. Entropy measures randomness of gray-scale levels. Correlation and Haralick's Correlation measured image linearity. Inertia measures the variance of image. Cluster Shade and Cluster Prominence measures the skewness of kurtosis.

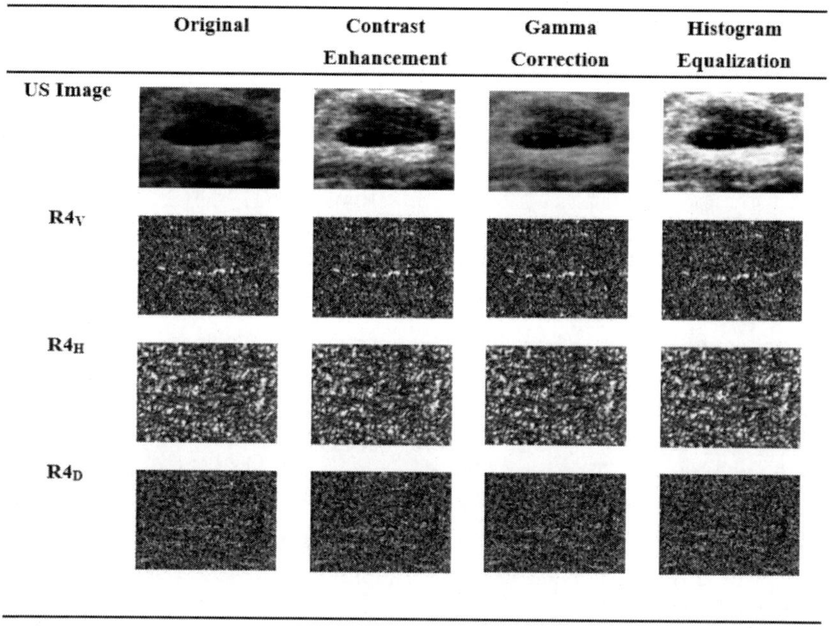

Figure 3. Images of original ultrasound B-mode image (US image) and ranklet transform image (R4V, R4H, R4D) undergoing contrast enhancement, gamma correction, and histogram equalization.

$p(i, j|d, \theta)$ is a probability of two neighbouring pixels at d distance and θ direction, one with gray-scale value i, and another with gray-scale value j. In this study, distance d is set to 1. Four directions were considered (θ = 0°, 45°, 90°, 135°).

$$Energy = \sum_i \sum_j p(i,j|d,\theta)^2 \tag{14}$$

$$Entropy = -\sum_i \sum_j p(i,j|d,\theta)\log(p(i,j|d,\theta)) \tag{15}$$

$$Correlation = \frac{\sum_i \sum_j (i-u_x)(j-u_y)p(i,j|d,\theta)}{\sigma_x \sigma_y} \tag{16}$$

$$Local\ Homogeneity = \sum_i \sum_j \frac{1}{1+(i-j)^2} p(i,j|d,\theta) \tag{17}$$

$$Inertia = \sum_i \sum_j (i-j)^2 p(i,j|d,\theta) \tag{18}$$

$$Cluster\ Shade = \sum_i \sum_j (i+j-u_x-u_y)^3 p(i,j|d,\theta) \tag{19}$$

$$Cluster\ Prominence = \sum_i \sum_j (i+j-u_x-u_y)^4 p(i,j|d,\theta) \tag{20}$$

$$Haralick's\ Correlation = \frac{\sum_i \sum_j (i \cdot j) p(i,j|d,\theta) - u_x u_y}{\sigma_x \sigma_y} \tag{21}$$

μ_x and μ_y are mean. σ_x and σ_y are standard deviation of the marginal distributions of $p(i, j|d, \theta)$.

$$u_x = \sum_i i \sum_j p(i,j|d,\theta), \quad u_y = \sum_j j \sum_i p(i,j|d,\theta) \tag{22}$$

$$\sigma_x^2 = \sum_i (i-u_x)^2 \sum_j p(i,j|d,\theta), \sigma_y^2 = \sum_j (j-u_y)^2 \sum_i p(i,j|d,\theta) \tag{23}$$

Both the tumor texture and speckle textures are extracted by using GLCM. In total, there are 240 features each for texture and speckle texture (3 orientations × 5 resolutions for ranklet transform × 8 GLCM-derived features × 2 average or standard deviation).

3.6. Results and Discussion

There are 480 features with half of texture and the other half of speckle features. The distribution of each features were assessed by Kolmogorov-Smirnov test. 186 of texture features and 181 speckle features were normally distributed. Depending on the distribution of each feature, Student's t-test or

Mann-Whitney U-test was used for pre-selection of statistically significant (p-value < 0.05) features into backward elimination of binary logistic regression model. As a result of the pre-selection, there were 46 texture features and 35 speckle features statistically significant in differentiating benign and malignant tumor. Through backward- stepwise- elimination of binary logistic regression model, 10 texture features and 11 speckle features remained in the model. The most commonly selected features were from R32H ranklet transform images. They are entropy average, correlation standard deviation, cluster prominence standard deviation, and Haralick correlation average. It is not by chance that resolution of 32 is also the highest resolution used in this study. During ranklet transform, a higher resolution takes into consideration of more pixels when assigning rank based on intensity of the crop. Such finding renders a follow up question of what is the optimized resolution for texture analysis in ultrasonography. What is the tumor biology basis of the heterogeneity in ultrasonography image? These questions are to be addressed in carefully designed studies.

Table 4. Assessment of ranklet transform performance on texture and speckles features by Chi-Square test

	Tumor texture	Tumor texture (ranklet)	p-value	Speckle texture	Speckle texture (ranklet)	p-value
Accuracy	58% (40/69)	80% (55/69)	0.0058*	62% (43/69)	83% (57/69)	0.0076*
Sensitivity	38% (8/21)	76% (16/21)	0.0126*	33% (7/21)	71% (15/21)	0.0134
Specificity	67% (32/48)	81% (39/48)	0.1035	75% (36/48)	88% (42/48)	0.1167
PPV	33% (8/24)	64% (16/25)	0.0318*	37% (7/19)	71% (15/21)	0.0281*
NPV	71% (32/45)	89% (39/44)	0.0396*	72% (36/50)	88% (42/48)	0.057
Az	0.58	0.83	0.0009*	0.56	0.80	0.02*

PPV: positive predictive value
NPV: negative predictive value
Az: Area under ROC curve
* p-value < 0.05

The nature of each tumor case is predicted based on the 10 texture features and 11 speckle features in binary logistic regression model. Comparing the prediction with biopsy-proven result, 5 performance indices including accuracy, sensitivity, specificity, positive predictive value (PPV), negative predictive value (NPV); were calculated and shown in Table 4. Chi-Square test was utilized for evaluation of statistical significance. Ranklet transform increase the all 5 performance indices of prediction in both texture and speckle features. They were statistically significant in most indices, except NPV of speckle features, specificity of texture and speckle features. Receiver Operating Characteristic (ROC) curve was drawn for various sensitivity and specificity. Area under the ROC curve was calculated. Ranklet transform significantly improve the prediction power of texture and speckle features.

4. Genomic Correlation of MRI-Based Tumor Phenotype in Invasive Breast Carcinoma

4.1. Data Acquisitions

This retrospective study involved 91 breast cancer cases. Genomic data of these cases including 20,531 gene expressions, 19,950 copy number variations, 142 protein expressions, 1,046 miRNA expression, and 3,734 somatic mutations were downloaded from The Cancer Genome Atlas (TCGA) public domain. Most of the genomic data were available for 91 cases, except there were only 62 data sets for protein expressions. DCE-MRI images were downloaded from The Cancer Imaging Archive (TCIA) [55]. 38 radiomic features were extracted from primary breast tumors in DCE-MRI image. These features can be classified into size, shape, margin, enhancement texture, kinetics, and variance kinetics.

The 91 breast cancer cases are composed of 22 pathological stage I, 58 stage II, and 11 stage III sample. There were no signs of metastasis in MRI images. 77 cases are ER(+), 72 are PR(+), and 19 are HER2(+).

4.2. Radiomics Features

There are 38 radiomic features in 6 categories. Refer to supplemental section of original article [21] for equation and description of the following features:

1. Size phenotypes are (1) tumor volume, (2) surface area, (3) maximum linear size, and (4) effective diameter. The effective diameter is the diameter of sphere with the same tumor volume.
2. Shape phenotypes are (5) sphericity, (6) irregularity, and (7) surface-to-volume ratio. Sphericity is the ratio between volume of lesion

within a sphere (with effective diameter) and tumor volume. Irregularity represents a ratio of effective area and surface area.

3. Morphology phenotypes are (8) margin sharpness, (9) variance of margin sharpness and (10) variance of radial gradient histogram.
4. Enhancement texture characterizes texture of tumor on first post-contrast image. GLCM is the basis of these features. These radiomic features are (11) energy, (12) contrast, (13) correlation, (14) entropy, (15) variance, (16) difference entropy, (17) different variance, (18) inverse difference moment, (19) sum average, (20) sum entropy, (21) sum variance, (22, 23) information measure of correlation, and (24) maximum correlation coefficient.
5. Kinetic curve assessment captures the uptake and washout of contrast media in tumor during dynamic image in series. These features are (25) maximum enhancement, (26) time to peak, (27) uptake time, (28) washout rate, (29) curve shape index, (30) enhancement at first post-contrast time-point, (31) signal enhancement ratio, (32) volume of most enhancing voxels, (33) total rate variation, and (34) normalized total rate variation.
6. Enhancement-variance kinetics represents the spatial variance of enhancement at time course. These features are (35) maximum variance of enhancement, (36) time to peak at maximum variance, (37) enhancement variance increasing rate, and (38) enhancement variance decreasing rate.

4.3. Results and Discussion

The association between genomic features and radiomic phenotypes including tumor size, shape, morphology, enhancement textures, kinetic curve assessments, and enhancement-variance kinetics were investigated. Linear regression analysis was performed to identify connection of radiomic features to mutated genes, miRNA, and protein expression. Reverse Phase Protein Array (RPPA) was utilized to measure 142 protein expression levels related to breast cancer. Gene expression was studied in groups according to known molecular biology pathways documented in Kyoto Encyclopedia of Genes and Genomes (KEGG) database [56] by Gene-Set Enrichment Analysis (GSEA) [57]. P-value of < 0.05 is regarded as statistically significant. Fischer's exact test was applied to the number of significant associations on each radiomic feature groups to investigate if certain radiomic phenotypes more likely to be associated with particular genomic features.

miRNA expressions are associated with tumor size and enhancement textures. 92.3% of miRNA expressions are correlated to 3 of the 4 tumor size phenotypes including tumor volume, surface area, and effective diameter, but not maximal tumor diameter. This leads to a general hypothesis that miRNA is associated with tumor growth, but it may not be related to tumor margin irregularity. Copy Number Variations of pathways are only associated with tumor size phenotypes and enhancement variance kinetics. Protein expressions are only correlated to tumor size phenotypes and morphological phenotypes.

Transcriptional activities of pathways are associated with all 6 types of radiomic phenotypes. In particular, 97.7% of pathway transcriptional activities are positively associated with all 4 phenotypes of tumor size including tumor volume, surface area, maximum linear size, and effective diameter. In addition, most of the pathway transcriptional activities are negatively associated with 2 of the 3 morphology phenotypes including margin sharpness and variance of radial gradient histogram. The pathway transcriptional activities are also found to be positively associated with 2 of the 3 shape phenotypes including irregularity and surface to volume ratio. Hence, up-regulation of many transcriptional pathways is associated to tumor growth, uneven tumor margin, and irregular shape, a potential sign of local invasiveness and aggressiveness. Tumor size phenotypes are correlated to up-regulation of transcriptional pathways including DNA replication, cell cyle, P53, base excision repair, mismatch repair, and cell adhesion molecules. The role of cell adhesion molecules in Epithelial-Mesenchymal Transition (EMT) is well characterized. Gap-junctions and cell adhesion protein expression decreases and disrupts cell-cell and cell-extracellular matrix interaction. Loss-of-function of cell adhesion molecules is associated with malignancy, local invasion, and metastasis. In this study, cell adhesion gene expression is correlated with larger tumor size (all four tumor size phenotypes), tumor margin irregularity (positive correlation with irregularity and negative with sphericity), and tissue perfusion (maximum enhancement, enhancement at the first post-contrast time point, and uptake time). Protein expression of P-cadherin confirms positively associated with tumor size (tumor volume, surface area, and effective diameter). Although it is feasible to explain the relation between tumor growth with DNA replication, and cell cycle under the context of cell proliferation, the explanation of other pathways is not straightforward. For example, p53 is a tumor suppressive gene with loss-of-function resulted in tumorigenesis. But, p53 gene mutation is absent in all cases of this database. Instead, p53 is positively associated with tumor margin irregularity, tumor size, and tissue perfusion. Some of the important role on gene expression that is well characterized in population is not seen in this study. For example, BRCA gene is well characterized in breast cancer aggressiveness. But, the role of this gene is not shown in this study. Hence, there is no simple explanation to these presence and absence of correlations.

This study uses genomic data acquired from a single tissue biopsy. The diagnostic power of biopsy in representing the characteristics of the whole tumor has always been questioned. In order to better represent the tumor, multiple biopsies can be attained with accurate location specification. This will allow a more direct correlation of radiomic phenotypes with genomic features. Although there are only 38 radiomic phenotypes in this study, the redundancy of these phenotypes in each category is always a question. In order to ensure the representative power of phenotypes, features correlation analysis such as Principle Component Analysis (PCA) could be performed and select only 1 highly correlated phenotype in each group. When attempting to explain association between radiomic phenotypes and genomic features, the number of sample could limit the connection with known molecular pathways. The genomic diversity in human species is great. It took a huge sample size to identify a particular pathological gene in a disease. Nonetheless, it provided a pilot study to such extensive correlation and made the association result publicly available for further development.

5. CONCLUSION

The correlation of radiomic phenotypes and genomic features offers a unique perspective for investigation of cancer and an opportunity to extend CAD system into cancer biology. A better understanding of radiomic phenotypes on disease model and genomic association will help selection of better features for disease prediction or characterization. The establishment of consensus and robust methodology will foster a reproducible and comprehensible CAD system. A CAD system that will not only making prediction or diagnosiss but also justifying how decision is reached with mechanism basis. By selecting appropriate algorithm for image preprocessing, the representative power of radiomic features will be improved. A more precise and accurate CAD system will be build.

REFERENCES

[1] Siegel, RL; Miller, KD; Jemal, A. "Cancer statistics, 2015," *CA Cancer J Clin*, 65, 5-29, (2015).

[2] Hoerger, TJ; Ekwueme, DU; Miller, JW; Uzunangelov, V; Hall, IJ; Segel, J; Royalty, J; Gardner, JG; Smith, JL; Li, C. "Estimated Effects of the National Breast and Cervical Cancer Early Detection Program on Breast Cancer Mortality," *American Journal of Preventive Medicine*, 40, 397-404, (2010).

[3] Smart, CR; Byrne, C; Smith, RA; Garfinkel, L; Letton, AH; Dodd, GD; Beahrs, OH. "Twenty-year follow-up of the breast cancers diagnosed during the Breast Cancer Detection Demonstration Project," *CA: A Cancer Journal for Clinicians*, 47, 134-149, (1997).

[4] Tabár, L; Vitak, B; Chen, HH; Duffy, SW; Yen, MF; Chiang, CF; Krusemo, UB; Tot, T; Smith, RA. "THE SWEDISH TWO-COUNTY TRIAL TWENTY YEARS LATER: Updated Mortality Results and New Insights from Long-Term Follow-up," *RADIOL. CLIN. NORTH AM.*, 38, 625-651, (2000).

[5] Tabár, L; Vitak, B; Chen, HHT; Yen, MF; Duffy, SW; Smith, RA. "Beyond randomized controlled trials," *Cancer*, 91, 1724-1731, (2001).

[6] Feig, SA. "Effect of service screening mammography on population mortality from breast carcinoma," *Cancer*, 95, 451-457, (2002).

[7] Humphrey, LL; Helfand, M; Chan, BKS; Woolf, SH. "Breast Cancer Screening: A Summary of the Evidence for the U.S. Preventive Services Task Force," *Annals of Internal Medicine*, 137, 347-360, (2002).

[8] Kolb, TM; Lichy, J; Newhouse, JH. "Occult cancer in women with dense breasts: detection with screening US--diagnostic yield and tumor characteristics," *Radiology*, 207, 191-199, (1998).

[9] Gordon, PB; Goldenberg, SL. "Malignant breast masses detected only by ultrasound. A retrospective review," *Cancer*, 76, 626-630, (1995).

[10] Berg, WA; Gilbreath, PL. "Multicentric and Multifocal Cancer: Whole-Breast US in Preoperative Evaluation," *Radiology*, 214, 59-66, (2000).

[11] Kaplan, SS. "Clinical Utility of Bilateral Whole-Breast US in the Evaluation of Women with Dense Breast Tissue," *Radiology*, 221, 641-649, (2001).

[12] Buchberger, W; Niehoff, A; Obrist, P; DeKoekkoek-Doll, P; Dünser, M. "Clinically and mammographically occult breast lesions: Detection and classification with high-resolution sonography," Seminars in Ultrasound, *CT and MRI*, 21, 325-336, (2000).

[13] Kashikura, Y; Nakayama, R; Hizukuri, A; Noro, A; Nohara, Y; Nakamura, T; Ito, M; Kimura, H; Yamashita, M; Hanamura, N; Ogawa, T. "Improved Differential Diagnosis of Breast Masses on Ultrasonographic Images with a Computer-Aided Diagnosis Scheme for Determining Histological Classifications," *Academic Radiology*, 20, 471-477, (2013).

[14] Drukker, K; Giger, ML; Metz, CE. "Robustness of Computerized Lesion Detection and Classification Scheme across Different Breast US Platforms," *Radiology*, 237, 834-840, (2005).

[15] Moon, WK; Lo, CM; Cho, N; Chang, JM; Huang, CS; Chen, JH; Chang, RF. "Computer-aided diagnosis of breast masses using quantified BI-RADS findings," *Computer Methods and Programs in Biomedicine*, 111, 84-92, (2013).

[16] Lo, CM; Chang, YC; Yang, YW; Huang, CS; Chang, RF. "Quantitative breast mass classification based on the integration of B-mode features and strain features in elastography," *Comput Biol Med*, 64, 91-100, (2015).

[17] Moon, WK; Lo, CM; Chang, JM; Huang, CS; Chen, JH; Chang, RF. "Quantitative Ultrasound Analysis for Classification of BI-RADS Category 3 Breast Masses," *Journal of Digital Imaging*, 26, 1091-1098, (2013).

[18] Lo, CM; Moon, WK; Huang, CS; Chen, JH; Yang, MC; Chang, RF. "Intensity-Invariant Texture Analysis for Classification of BI-RADS Category 3 Breast Masses," *Ultrasound Med Biol*, 41, 2039-2048, (2015).

[19] Haralick, RM; Shanmugam, K; Dinstein, IH. "Textural Features for Image Classification," Systems, Man and Cybernetics, *IEEE Transactions on SMC-3*, 610-621, (1973).

[20] Masotti, M; Lanconelli, N; Campanini, R. "Computer-aided mass detection in mammography: False positive reduction via gray-scale invariant ranklet texture features," *Medical Physics*, 36, 311-316, (2009).

[21] Zhu, Y; Li, H; Guo, W; Drukker, K; Lan, L; Giger, ML; Ji, Y. "Deciphering Genomic Underpinnings of Quantitative MRI-based Radiomic Phenotypes of Invasive Breast Carcinoma," *Sci Rep*, 5, 17787, (2015).

[22] Wibmer, A; Hricak, H; Gondo, T; Matsumoto, K; Veeraraghavan, H; Fehr, D; Zheng, J; Goldman, D; Moskowitz, C; Fine, SW; Reuter, VE; Eastham, J; Sala, E; Vargas, HA. "Haralick texture analysis of prostate MRI: utility for differentiating non-cancerous prostate from prostate cancer and differentiating prostate cancers with different Gleason scores," *European Radiology*, 25, 2840-2850, (2015).

[23] Jamshidi, N; Diehn, M; Bredel, M; Kuo, MD. "Illuminating Radiogenomic Characteristics of Glioblastoma Multiforme through Integration of MR Imaging, Messenger RNA Expression, and DNA Copy Number Variation," *Radiology*, 270, 1-2, (2013).

[24] Karlo, CA; Paolo, PLD; Chaim, J; Hakimi, AA; Ostrovnaya, I; Russo, P; Hricak, H; Motzer, R; Hsieh, JJ; Akin, O. "Radiogenomics of Clear Cell Renal Cell Carcinoma: Associations between CT Imaging Features and Mutations," *Radiology*, 270, 464-471, (2014).

[25] Aerts, HJ; Velazquez, ER; Leijenaar, RT; Parmar, C; Grossmann, P; Carvalho, S; Bussink, J; Monshouwer, R; Haibe-Kains, B; Rietveld, D; Hoebers, F; Rietbergen, MM; Leemans, CR; Dekker, A; Quackenbush, J; Gillies, RJ; Lambin, P. "Decoding tumour phenotype by noninvasive imaging using a quantitative radiomics approach," *Nat Commun*, 5, 4006, (2014).

[26] Suri, JS. *Advances in diagnostic and therapeutic ultrasound imaging.*, (Artech House, 2008).

[27] Deriche, R. "Fast algorithms for low-level vision," Pattern Analysis and Machine Intelligence, *IEEE Transactions on*, 12, 78-87, (1990).

[28] Moon, WK; Chang, SC; Huang, CS; Chang, RF. "Breast tumor classification using fuzzy clustering for breast elastography," *Ultrasound Med Biol*, 37, 700-708, (2011).

[29] Garra, BS; Cespedes, EI; Ophir, J; Spratt, SR; Zuurbier, RA; Magnant, CM; Pennanen, MF. "Elastography of breast lesions: initial clinical results," *Radiology*, 202, 79-86, (1997).

[30] Lo, CM; Chen, YP; Chang, YC; Lo, C; Huang, CS; Chang, RF. "Computer-Aided Strain Evaluation for Acoustic Radiation Force Impulse Imaging of Breast Masses," *Ultrasonic Imaging*, 36, 151-166, (2014).

[31] Kallel, F; Ophir, J. "A Least-Squares Strain Estimator for Elastography," *Ultrasonic Imaging*, 19, 195-208, (1997).

[32] Varghese, T; Ophir, J. "A theoretical framework for performance characterization of elastography: the strain filter," *Ultrasonics, Ferroelectrics, and Frequency Control, IEEE Transactions on*, 44, 164-172, (1997).

[33] Davnall, F; Yip, CS; Ljungqvist, G; Selmi, M; Ng, F; Sanghera, B; Ganeshan, B; Miles, KA; Cook, GJ; Goh, V. "Assessment of tumor heterogeneity: an emerging imaging tool for clinical practice?," *Insights Imaging*, 3, 573-589, (2012).

[34] Burnside, ES; Hall, TJ; Sommer, AM; Hesley, GK; Sisney, GA; Svensson, WE. "Differentiating Benign from Malignant Solid Breast Masses with US Strain Imaging," *Radiology*, 245, 401-410, (2007).

[35] Jung, HJ; Hahn, SY; Choi, HY; Park, SH; Park, HK. "Breast sonographic elastography using an advanced breast tissue-specific imaging preset: Initial clinical results," *J. Ultrasound Med.*, 31, 273-280, (2012).

[36] Stachs, A; Hartmann, S; Stubert, J;. Dieterich, M; Martin, A; Kundt, G; Reimer, T; Gerber, B. "Differentiating between malignant and benign breast masses: Factors limiting sonoelastographic strain ratio," *Ultraschall Med.*, 34, 131-136 (2013).

[37] Leong, LC; Sim, LS; Lee, YS; Ng, FC; Wan, CM; Fook-Chong, SM; Jara-Lazaro, AR; Tan, PH. "A prospective study to compare the diagnostic performance of breast elastography versus conventional breast ultrasound," *Clin Radiol*, 65, 887-894, (2010).

[38] Xu, H; Rao, M; Varghese, T; Sommer, A; Baker, S; Hall, TJ; Sisney, GA; Burnside, ES. "Axial-shear strain imaging for differentiating benign and malignant breast masses," *Ultrasound Med Biol*, 36, 1813-1824, (2010).

[39] Xu, H; Varghese, T; Jiang, J; Zagzebski, JA. "*In Vivo* Classification of Breast Masses Using Features Derived From Axial-Strain and Axial-Shear Images," *Ultrasonic Imaging*, 34, 222-236, (2012).

[40] Itoh, A; Ueno, E; Tohno, E; Kamma, H; Takahashi, H; Shiina, T; Yamakawa, M; Matsumura, T. "Breast disease: clinical application of US elastography for diagnosis," *Radiology*, 239, 341-350, (2006).

[41] Céspedes, I; Ophir, J; Ponnekanti, H; Maklad, N. "Elastography: Elasticity Imaging Using Ultrasound with Application to Muscle and Breast *in Vivo*," *Ultrasonic Imaging*, 15, 73-88, (1993).

[42] Thittai, AK; Yamal, JM; Mobbs, LM; Kraemer-Chant, CM; Chekuri, S; Garra, BS; Ophir, J. "Axial-shear strain elastography for breast lesion classification: further results from *in vivo* data," *Ultrasound Med Biol*, 37, 189-197, (2011).

[43] Thitaikumar, A; Ophir, J. "Effect of lesion boundary conditions on axial strain elastograms: a parametric study," *Ultrasound Med Biol*, 33, 1463-1467, (2007).

[44] Nie, K; Chen, JH; Chan, S; Chau, MKI; Yu, HJ; Bahri, S; Tseng, T; Nalcioglu, O; Su, MY. "Development of a quantitative method for analysis of breast density based on three-dimensional breast MRI," *Medical Physics*, 35, 5253-5262, (2008).

[45] Dunn, JC. "A Graph Theoretic Analysis of Pattern Classification via Tamura's Fuzzy Relation," Systems, Man and Cybernetics, *IEEE Transactions on SMC-4*, 310-313, (1974).

[46] Bezdek, JC; Ehrlich, R; Full, W. "FCM: The fuzzy c-means clustering algorithm," *Computers and Geosciences*, 10, 191-203, (1984).

[47] Chuai-Aree, S; Lursinsap, C; Sophasathit, P; Siripant, S. "FUZZY C-MEAN: A STATISTICAL FEATURE CLASSIFICATION OF TEXT AND IMAGE SEGMENTATION METHOD," International Journal of Uncertainty, *Fuzziness and Knowledge-Based Systems*, 09, 661-671, (2001).

[48] Nie, K; Chen, JH; Yu, HJ; Chu, Y; Nalcioglu, O; Su, MY. "Quantitative analysis of lesion morphology and texture features for diagnostic prediction in breast MRI," *Acad Radiol*, 15, 1513-1525, (2008).

[49] Tuthill, T; Sperry, R; Parker, K. "Deviations from Rayleigh statistics in ultrasonic speckle," *Ultrasonic imaging*, 10, 81-89, (1988).

[50] Moon, WK; Lo, CM; Chang, JM; Huang, CS; Chen, JH; Chang, RF. "Computer-aided classification of breast masses using speckle features of automated breast ultrasound images," *Medical Physics*, 39, 6465-6473, (2012).

[51] Moon, WK; Lo, CM; Huang, CS; Chen, JH; Chang, RF. "Computer-Aided Diagnosis Based on Speckle Patterns in Ultrasound Images," *Ultrasound in Medicine and Biology*, 38, 1251-1261, (2012).

[52] Berg, WA; Blume, JD; Cormack, JB; et al., "Combined screening with ultrasound and mammography vs mammography alone in women at elevated risk of breast cancer," *JAMA*, 299, 2151-2163, (2008).

[53] Chung-Ming, L; Rong-Tai, C; Yeun-Chung, C; Ya-Wen, Y; Ming-Jen, H; Chiun-Sheng, H; Ruey-Feng, C. "Multi-Dimensional Tumor Detection in Automated Whole Breast Ultrasound Using Topographic Watershed," *Medical Imaging, IEEE Transactions on*, 33, 1503-1511, (2014).

[54] Min-Chun, Y; Woo Kyung, M; Wang, YCF; Min Sun, B; Chiun-Sheng, H; Jeon-Hor, C; Ruey-Feng, C. "Robust Texture Analysis Using Multi-Resolution Gray-Scale Invariant Features for Breast Sonographic Tumor Diagnosis," *Medical Imaging, IEEE Transactions on*, 32, 2262-2273, (2013).

[55] Clark, K; Vendt, B; Smith, K; Freymann, J; Kirby, J; Koppel, P; Moore, S; Phillips, S; Maffitt, D; Pringle, M; Tarbox, L; Prior, F. "The Cancer Imaging Archive (TCIA): Maintaining and Operating a Public Information Repository," *Journal of Digital Imaging*, 26, 1045-1057, (2013).

[56] Kanehisa, M; Goto, S; Sato, Y; Furumichi, M; Tanabe, M. "KEGG for integration and interpretation of large-scale molecular data sets," *Nucleic Acids Research*, 40, D109-D114, (2012).

[57] Subramanian, A; Tamayo, P; Mootha, VK; Mukherjee, S; Ebert, BL; Gillette, MA; Paulovich, A; Pomeroy, SL; Golub, TR; Lander, ES; Mesirov, JP. "Gene set enrichment analysis: a knowledge-based approach for interpreting genome-wide expression profiles," *Proc Natl Acad Sci U S A*, 102, 15545-15550, (2005).

BIOGRAPHICAL SKETCHES

Name: Chung-Ming Lo

Affiliation: Taipei Medical University

Education: Ph.D. Department of Computer Science and Information Engineering, National Taiwan University

Research and Professional Experience: Assistant Professor, Taipei Medical University

Professional Appointments: Medical Image Processing

Honors:

- 2015-12th National Innovation Award
- 2015-MOST Reward of Excellent Faculty Recruitment
- 2014-MOST Postdoc Academic Publication Award
- 2014-International Federation for Medical and Biological Engineering, Young Investigator Award
- 2013-26th IPPR CVGIP Excellent Paper Award

Publications Last Three Years:

1. Chung-Ming Lo, Siwa Chan, Ya-Wen Yang, Yeun-Chung Chang, Chiun-Sheng Huang*, Yi-Sheng Jou, and Ruey-Feng Chang* (2015, Dec). Feasibility Testing: Three-dimensional Tumor Mapping in Different Orientations of Automated Breast Ultrasound. Ultrasound in Medicine and Biology. (Accepted). (SCI, IF=2.214, 5/31, ACOUSTICS)

2. Chung-Ming Lo, Yi-Chen Lai, Yi-Hong Chou*, and Ruey-Feng Chang* (2015, Sep). Quantitative Breast Lesion Classification Based on Multichannel Distributions in Shear-wave Imaging. Computer Methods and Programs in Biomedicine, 122(3), 354-361. (SCI, IF=1.897, 15/102, COMPUTER SCIENCE, THEORY and METHODS).
3. Chung-Ming Lo, Yeun-Chung Chang, Ya-Wen Yang, Chiun-Sheng Huang*, Ruey-Feng Chang* (2015, Jun). Quantitative Breast Mass Classification Based on The Integration of B-mode Features and Strain Features in Elastography. Computers in Biology and Medicine, 64, 91-100. (SCI, IF= 1.240, 49/85, BIOLOGY)
4. Ruey-Feng Chang, Yu-Ling Hou, Chung-Ming Lo, Chiun-Sheng Huang, JeonHor Chen, Won Hwa Kim, Jung Min Chang, Min Sun Bae, Woo Kyung Moon* (2015, Aug). Quantitative Analysis of Breast Echotexture Patterns in Automated Breast Ultrasound Images. Medical Physics, 42(8), 4566-4578. (SCI, IF=2.635, 38/125, RADIOLOGY, NUCLEAR MEDICINE and MEDICAL IMAGING).
5. Chung-Ming Lo, Woo Kyung Moon*, Chiun-Sheng Huang, Jeon-Hor Chen, Min-Chun Yang, Ruey-Feng Chang* (2015, Jul). Intensity-Invariant Texture Analysis for Classification of BI-RADS Category 3 Breast Masses. Ultrasound in Medicine and Biology. 41(7). 2039-2048. (SCI, IF=2.214, 5/31, ACOUSTICS).

6. Woo Kyung Moon, Yao-Sian Huang, Chung-Ming Lo, Chiun-Sheng Huang, Min Sun Bae, Won Hwa Kim, Jeon-Hor Chen, Ruey-Feng Chang* (2015, June). Computer-aided Diagnosis for Distinguishing between Triple-negative Breast Cancer and Fibroadenomas Based on Ultrasound Texture Features. Medical Physics, 42(6), 3024-3035. (SCI, IF=2.635, 38/125, RADIOLOGY, NUCLEAR MEDICINE and MEDICAL IMAGING).
7. Chung-Ming Lo, Rong-Tai Chen, Yeun-Chung Chang, Ya-Wen Yang, Ming-Jen Hung, Chiun-Sheng Huang*, Ruey-Feng Chang* (2014, Jul). Multi-dimensional Tumor Detection in Automated Whole Breast Ultrasound using Topographic Watershed. IEEE TRANSACTIONS ON MEDICAL IMAGING, 33(7), 1503-11. (SCI, IF=3.390, 18/249, ENGINEERING, ELECTRICAL and ELECTRONIC).
8. Chung-Ming Lo, Yen-Po Chen, Yeun-Chung Chang, Chiao Lo, Chiun-Sheng Huang*, Ruey-Feng Chang* (2014, Jun). Computer-Aided Strain Evaluation for Acoustic Radiation Force Impulse Imaging of Breast Masses. Ultrasonic Imaging, 36(3), 151-166. (SCI, IF=0.912, 16/31, Acoustics).
9. Woo Kyung Moon, Chung-Ming Lo, Rong-Tai Chen, Yi-Wei Shen, Jung Min Chang, Chiun-Sheng Huang, Jeon-Hor Chen, Wei-Wen Hsu, Ruey-Feng Chang* (2014, Apr). Tumor Detection in Automated Breast Ultrasound Images using Quantitative Tissue Clustering. Medical Physics, 41(4), 042901. (SCI, IF=2.635, 38/125, RADIOLOGY, NUCLEAR MEDICINE and MEDICAL IMAGING).
10. Woo Kyung Moon, Chung-Ming Lo, Jin-Mo Goo, Min Sun Bae, Jung Min Chang, Chiun-Sheng Huang, Jeon-Hor Chen, Violeta Ivanova, Ruey-Feng Chang* (2014, Mar). Quantitative Analysis for Breast Density Estimation in Low Dose Chest CT Scans. Journal of Medical Systems, 38(3), 1-9. (SCI, IF=2.213, 7/24, MEDICAL INFORMATICS).
11. Woo Kyung Moon, Chung-Ming Lo, Jung Min Chang, Chiun-Sheng Huang, Jeon-Hor Chen, Ruey-Feng Chang* (2013, Dec). Quantitative Ultrasound Analysis for Classification of BI-RADS Category 3 Breast Masses. Journal of Digital Imaging, 26(6), 1091-1098. (SCI, IF=1.190, 95/125, RADIOLOGY, NUCLEAR MEDICINE and MEDICAL IMAGING).
12. Woo Kyung Moon, Chung-Ming Lo, Jung Min Chang, Min Sun Bae, Won Hwa Kim, Chiun-Sheng Huang, Jeon-Hor Chen, Ming-Hong

Kuo, Ruey-Feng Chang* (2013, Oct). Rapid Breast Density Analysis of Partial Volumes of Automated Breast Ultrasound Images. Ultrasonic Imaging, 35(4), 333-343. (SCI, IF=0.912, 16/31, Acoustics).

13. Woo Kyung Moon, Chung-Ming Lo (co-first), Nariya Choa, Jung Min Changa, Chiun-Sheng Huang, Jeon-Hor Chen, Ruey-Feng Chang* (2013, Jul). Computer-aided Diagnosis of Breast Masses using Quantified BI-RADS Findings. Computer Methods and Programs in Biomedicine, 111(1), 84-92. (SCI, IF=1.897, 15/102, COMPUTER SCIENCE, THEORY and METHODS).

Ng Kee Koon

Affiliation: Taipei Medical University

Education: M.D. Taipei Medical University

Research and Professional Experience: Research Assistant, Taipei Medical University

Honors:

Tau Beta Pi (National Honor Society of Engineering)

Omega Chi Epsilon (National Honor Society of Chemical Engineering)

In: Horizons in Cancer Research. Volume 63 ISBN: 978-1-53610-013-6
Editor: Hiroto S. Watanabe

Chapter 4

DENDRITIC CELLS CROSS TALK WITH CYTOMEGALOVIRUS PP65-SPECIFIC CYTOTOXIC T CELLS, Vγ9γδT CELLS, AND INVARIANT NKT CELLS IN PATIENTS WITH GLIOBLASTOMA MULTIFORME

Mie Nieda[1], Hiroshi Terunuma[1], Yuuta Eiraku[1], Xuewen Deng[1] and Andrew J. Nicol[2]
[1]Biotherpy Institute of Japan, Kouto-ku, Tokyo, Japan
[2]University of Queensland; Greenslopes Private Hospital, Brisbane, Australia

ABSTRACT

Dendritic cell (DC)-based tumor vaccines called DC therapy are being explored as a promising therapeutic option to stimulate immune responses that recognize and selectively eliminate malignant cells. For successful DC therapy, it is crucial to marshal and orchestrate a vast array of effector cells. These cells include *adaptive immune cells* such as tumor-antigen-specific CD8+ T cells and CD4+ helper T cells, *innate immune cells* such as γδT cells and NK cells, and *innate/adaptive immune cells,* invariant NKT cells (iNKT) in which DCs play a pivotal role in bridging innate and adaptive immunities. In this study, we demonstrate in patients with glioblastoma multiforme (GBM) that copulsing cytomegalovirus derived peptide, pp65 (CMVpp65-peptide)-pulsed IFN-DCs with zoledronate (Z) and α-galactosylceramide (α-GalCer; G) efficiently induce CMVpp65-specific cytotoxic CD8+ T cells through Vγ9γδT cell and iNKT cell expansion. The IFN-DCs derived from patients with GBM used in this study express higher levels of CD56, CD14, and CD36 and lower levels of PDL1 and PDL2 than the most commonly used mature IL-4DCs. The expression of the lymph-node-homing receptor CCR7 on IFN-DCs was up-regulated following their culture with the peptide, Z, and G. In the supernatant of co-culture of lymphocytes and autologous IFN-DCs in the presence of the peptide, Z, and G, higher amounts of Th1 cytokines such as IFNγ and TNFα which are favorable for induction of cytotoxic T cell , higher amounts of IL-18, which up-regulate DC function, and lower amounts of IL-6, which down-regulate DC function, were detected than in the supernatant of co-culture of lymphocytes with autologous IFN-DCs in the presence of the peptide alone. Multifunctional T cells including HLA-A*0201-specific CMVpp65-specific CD8+T cells, Vγ9γδT cells, and iNKT cells efficiently kill HLA-A*0201-positive GBM tumor cell line.

Keywords: human, CMVpp65-specific cytotoxic CD8+ T, glioma multiform, zoledronate, α-galactosylceramide

INTRODUCTION

Dendritic cell (DC)-based tumor vaccines called DC-therapy are being explored as a promising therapeutic option to stimulate immune responses that recognize and selectively eliminate malignant cells. DCs loaded with specific tumor antigens by various methods such as pulsing with peptides or proteins, the insertion of tumor-specific genes, and the transfection of tumor-specific RNAs have elicited antigen-specific antitumor responses in animal models, preclinical experiments, and clinical studies. However, following the administration of DCs pulsed with a tumor antigen, clinical responses are seen in a minority of patients [1, 2] because of weak induction of tumor-antigen-specific CD8+ T cells that can eradicate tumors.

For successful DC therapy, it is crucial to marshal and orchestrate a vast array of effector cells. These cells include adaptive immune cells such as tumor-antigen-specific CD8+ T cells and CD4+ helper T cells, innate immune cells such as γδT cells and NK cells, and innate/adaptive immune cells, invariant NKT (iNKT) cells. Together with these cells, DCs play a pivotal role in bridging innate and adaptive immunities. Thus, we and others have aimed to enhance the induction of tumor-antigen-specific CD8+T cells by DCs derived from patients with melanoma or multiple myeloma copulsed with a tumor antigen and zoledronate (Z), which activates and expands Vγ9γδT cells [3, 4]. Finally, it has been confirmed that the induction of tumor-antigen-specific CD8+T cells is amplified by the concurrent activation and proliferation of Vγ9γδT cells, which produce Th1 cytokines such as IFNγ and TNFα.

We aimed for a stronger induction of tumor-antigen-specific CD8+ T cells and speculated that further pulsing of DCs with α-galactosylceramide (G), which is a ligand of invariant iNKT cells, copulsed with Z and a tumor antigen may enhance tumor-antigen-specific CD8+ T cells through the expansion of iNKT cells, in addition to expansion of Vγ9γδT cells. A unique property of iNKT cells is their rapid secretion of cytokines in response to ligand-dependent stimulation. This leads to a rapid downstream activation of several other immune cells, including DCs and T cells [5], showing that iNKT cells may serve as an important bridge between innate and adaptive immunities. In humans, our in vivo study using DCs pulsed with G has demonstrated that the iNKT cells activated by G-pulsed DCs did bridge innate and adaptive immunities to induce the activation and proliferation of IFN-γ-producing CD8+ T cells following the activation and proliferation of iNKT and NK cells [6].

Taken together with these previous studies of DCs, Vγ9γδT cells, and iNKT cells, we highly expect that the infusion of DCs pulsed with a tumor antigen, Z, and G enhances the induction of tumor-antigen-specific CD8+ T cells. This enhanced induction occurs through the expansion of Vγ9γδT cells and iNKT in which Vγ9γδT cells and iNKT themselves also function as effector cells against tumors, resulting in a better clinical outcome.

In this study, we chose pp65, an antigen from a common herpes virus called cytomegalovirus (CMVpp65), in glioblastoma multiforme (GBM) as the tumor antigen [7]. GBM is an aggressive brain tumor in which cells specifically express pp65, making pp65 an attractive target for immunotherapy [7, 8]. Although the presence of CMV within malignant glioma has been confirmed by several laboratories, its relevance as an immunologic target in GBM has yet to be established [9, 10]. Despite conventional therapies such as surgery, radiation, and chemotherapy, treatment of patients with GBM is rarely curative, and conventional therapies are inherently nonspecific and damaging to surrounding normal tissues [11, 12]. Immunotherapies including DC therapy for patients with GBM provide a promising alternative owing to the intrinsic specificity and potentially long-lasting effects of immune activation with less toxicity.

We have recently demonstrated that in comparison with conventional mature IL-4DCs (mIL-4DCs) differentiated from monocytes obtained as adherent cells in the presence of GM-CSF, IL-4, and TNF-α, IFN-DCs expressing high levels of CD56 and CD14 which are differentiated from monocytes obtained as adherent cells in the presence of IFNα and GM-CSF more effectively induced melanoma-antigen-specific CD8+ T cells [13]. Thus, in this study we used IFN-DCs from GBM patients as a DC population.

Recently, various molecules that can modulate TCR signals have been identified [14, 15]. Multiple costimulatory and inhibitory interactions regulate T cell responses to antigen-presenting cells (APCs) such as DCs [16]. These responses can occur upon the initiation of T cell responses in lymph nodes, peripheral tissues, or tumors [17]. Many ligands bind to multiple receptors, some of which deliver costimulatory signals and others deliver inhibitory signals. These include, besides the well-known CD28 and CTLA-4, the recently described molecules PD-1, ICOS, and BTLA4. Except for BTLA4, all interact with B7 family ligands. Besides B7-1 and B7-2, PD-L1, PD-L2, ICOS-L, B7-H3, and B7-H4 have been identified so far [18-20]. In this study, we have focused on the expression levels of PD-L1 and PDL-2 on DCs, which are associated with the induction of tumor-antigen-specific T cells. We also assessed the involvement of PD-L1 and PD-L2 on tumor targets derived from GBM patients in tumor control.

The aims of this study were as follows:

1. To determine whether IFN-DCs derived from GBM patients and HDs can most extensively induce CMVpp65-specific CD8+ T cells, in addition to the expansion of Vγ9γδT cells and iNKT cells in the presence of the CMVpp65-peptide with Z plus G in comparison with the presence of the peptide alone, the peptide with Z, or the peptide with G
2. To determine whether the induction of effector cells including CMVpp65-specific CD8+ T cells by IFN-DCs in the presence of the CMVpp65-peptide with Z plus G is enhanced following the further addition of anti-PDL1 monoclonal antibody (mAb).
3. To determine whether effector T cells including CMVpp65-specific CD8+ T cells, Vγ9γδT cells, and iNKT cells efficiently kill GBM tumor cell line (T98G) [21] wherein the killing activity of the effector

T cells is enhanced following the further addition of an anti-PDL1 and/or anti-PDL2 mAb.

4. To determine various cytokines produced following the culture of lymphocytes with IFN-DCs in the presence of the CMVpp65-peptide with Z plus G, in comparison with IFN-DCs in the presence of the peptide alone.

MATERIALS AND METHODS

Flow Cytometry and Reagents

Surface phenotypes were determined using an Epics XL MCL (Beckman Coulter, CA). The following mAbs were purchased from Beckman Coulter: anti-CD3, anti-CD4, anti-CD8, anti-Vγ9TCR, anti-CD14, anti-CD16, anti-CD45, anti-CD54, anti-CD56, anti-CD69, anti-HLADR, anti-CD40, anti-CD80, anti-CD86, anti-CD36, mouse IgG1, mouse IgG2, and mouse IgG2b mAbs. Anti-HLA-AB and anti-CCR7 mAbs were purchased from Beckton Dickinson (San Jose, CA) and R & D System (Minneapolis, MN), respectively. Anti-TCR Vα24TCR and anti-TCR Vβ11mAbs were purchased from Beckman Coulter (France). Anti-human CD273 (PDL-2) and CD274 (PDL-1)mAbs were purchased from eBioscience (CA). Anti-human CD152 (CTLA-4) and CD279 (PD-1) mAbs were purchased from BioLegend (CA). All mAbs were conjugated with FITC, PE, APC, ECD, PC5, or PC7. Purified anti-human CD152 (CTLA-4), CD273 (PD-L2), CD274 (PD-L1), and CD279 (PD-1) mAbs were purchased from eBioscience (CA). Z was purchased from Novartis Pharmaceuticals (Switzerland) and G from Funakoshi Co., Ltd. (Japan).

Generation of IFN-DCs

PBMCs were isolated from healthy donors (HDs) and Patients (Pts) with GBM. The study was approved by the Research Ethics Committee of the Biotherapy Institute of Japan for HDs and the Research Ethics Committee of the Queendsland Institute of Medical Research, the University of Queendsland for Pts. All the subjects provided their written informed consent to use their

PBMCs for research purpose. For cell culture in this study, AIM-V medium (Invitrogen, Japan) containing 10% heat-inactivated human AB serum was used. PBMCs separated by density gradient centrifugation with Lymphoprep (Nycomed, Norway) were suspended in the medium and then incubated in a flask (Corning Incorporated, Japan) for 1 h at 37°C. After removing nonadherent cells, monocytes obtained as adherent cells were cultured in the medium containing GM-CSF (1000 U/mL; Primmune Inc., Japan) and IFNα (1000 U/mL; INTRON, MSD K.K., Japan) for 3 days to obtain IFN-DCs. Alternatively, adherent cells were cultured for 5 days in the medium containing GM-CSF (1000U/mL) and IL-4 (500U/ml) to obtain IL-4DCs. The cells were further cultured for 2 days in the presence of TNFα (10ng/mL: Peprotech Ltd., UK) to obtain mature IL-4DCs (mIL-4DCs).

Induction of Tumor-Antigen-Specific CD8+ T Cells by IFN-DCs

To investigate MHC-restricted immune responses mediated by CD8+ T cells, HLA-A*0101-restricted, CMVpp65-modified 11-mer synthetic peptides (YSEHPTFTSQY) and/or HLA-A*0201-restricted, CMVpp65-9-mer synthetic peptides (NLVPMVATV) (Proimmune) were used. Lymphocytes ($2x10^6$) as a nonadherent cell fraction were cultured with autologous IFN-DCs ($2x10^5$) under different conditions. The lymphocytes possessing HLA-A*0201 and/or HLA-A*0101 were cultured with autologous IFN-DCs in the presence of the HLA-A*0201 and/or HLA-A*0101-restriced CMVpp65-peptide (5 μg/mL) for 10–14 days. In some experiments, Z (0.1 μM) and/or G (100ng/mL) was added during the culture. The cultures were supplemented with 50U/mL IL-2 (Chiron Benelux B. V., The Netherlands) during the culture. The percentage of CMVpp65-specific CD8+T cells was assessed using PE-CMVpp65 pentamer (Proimmune) and FITC-anti-CD8 mAb (Beckton Dickinson).

Cytotoxicity Assay

The HLA-A*0201-positive T98G tumor cell line that was established from a patient with GBM was purchased from the American Type Culture Collection (VA, USA) and used as the target cells. Fluorochromasia cell-mediated cytotoxicity assay was carried out using Terascan VPC (Minerva Tech, Japan), as described previously [22].

Determination of Cytokine Production Following Culture of DCs with Autologous Lymphocytes

Supernatants from the culture of DCs with autologous lymphocytes in the presence of the CMVpp65-peptide alone or in the presence of the peptide with Z plus G were harvested on days 1, 2, and 3. The cytokine contents of supernatants were determined by ELISA. IL-1β, IL-6, IL-12p70, IL-18, IFNγ, TNFα, and TGFβ were measured using OptEIA sets purchased from Beckman Coulter and Bender MedSystem Diagnosis (Vienna, Australia).

Statistical Analysis

The *p* values were calculated using paired/two-tailed Student's *t*-test and considered significant at <0.05 and highly significant at <0.01.

RESULTS

Phenotypical Analysis of IFN-DCs Derived from Monocytes as Adherent Cells in the Presence of IFNα and GM-CSF

To characterize surface antigens on IFN-DCs in comparison with those on mIL-4DCs, IFN-DCs and mIL-4DCs were differentiated from adherent cells obtained from four Pts with GBM. As representative results from Pt1, IFN-DCs showed an almost identical phenotypic pattern to mIL-DCs expressing high levels of HLA-class I, HLA-DR, CD80, CD86, CD40, and CD54 (data not shown), except in terms of the expressions of CD56, CD14, CD36, CCR7, PDL1, and PDL2 (Figure 1a). That is, the expression levels of CD56, CD14, CD36, and CCR7 on IFN-DCs were significantly higher than those on mIL-4DCs and the expression levels of PDL1 and PDL2 were significantly lower than those on mIL-4DCs (Figure 1b). The expression level of the scavenger receptor CD36 on IFN-DCs was significantly higher than that on mIL-4DCs, suggesting that IFN-DCs have higher processing ability than mIL-4DCs. As representative results from Pt 3, the expression level of CCR7 on IFN-DCs was also significantly higher than that on mIL-4DCs and gradually increased following the addition of CMVpp65-peptide and the peptide with Z plus G, (Figure 2a). Notably, the expression level of CCR7 on IFN-DCs in the presence of CMVpp65-peptide significantly increased following further addition of Z and G (Figure 2b). These results suggest that IFN-DCs pulsed with CMVpp65-peptide, Z, and G have a higher migration activity to the lymph nodes, which is associated with the effective interaction of such pulsed IFN-DCs with T cells in the lymph nodes than IFN-DCs pulsed with the peptide alone. Furthermore, expression levels of PDL1 and PDL2 on IFN-DCs, which are considered to predominantly mediate inhibitory signals towards T cells [18] were lower than those on mIL-4DCs, indicating that IFN-DCs have a higher ability to expand T cells than mIL-4DCs.

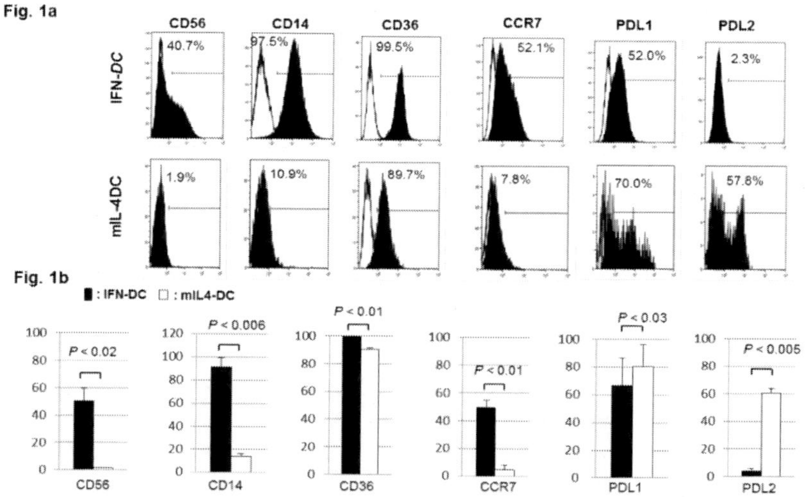

Figure 1. (a) Representative data on phenotypic patterns of CD56, CD14, CD36, CCR7, PDL1, and PDL2 on IFN-DCs and mIL-4DCs from Pt1 with glioblastoma multiform (GBM) (b) Statistical analysis of data from four Pts with GBM showed that the percentages of CD56+ cells, CD14+ cells, CD36+ cells, CCR7+ cells, PDL1+ cells, and PDL2+ cells among IFN-DCs were significantly higher than those among mIL-4DCs.

Extensive Induction of CMVpp65-Specific CD8+T Cells by IFN-DCs Derived from Patients with GBM in the Presence of the CMVpp65-Peptide with Z Plus G

The induction of CMVpp65-specific CD8+T cells by autologous IFN-DCs was examined under four different conditions: (1) IFN-DCs in the presence of the CMVpp65-peptide, (2) IFN-DCs in the presence of the CMVpp65-peptide with Z, (3) IFN-DCs in the presence of the CMVpp65-peptide with G, and (4) IFN-DCs in the presence of the CMVpp65-peptide with Z plus G. In the case of Pt1 possessing HLA-A*0201 and HLA-A*0101, after culture for 10 days, IFN-DCs most extensively induced CMVpp65-specific CD8+ T cells in the presence of the CMVpp65-peptide with Z plus G, in addition to Vγ9γδT cells and iNKT cells in the presence of the HLA-A*0101-restricted peptide (Table 1) and HLA-A*0201-restricted peptide (Table 2) and the induction ability of CMVpp65-specific CD8+ T cells by the HLA-A*0201-restricted peptide was higher than that by the HLA-A*0101-restricted peptide (Tables 1 and 2).

Fig. 2a

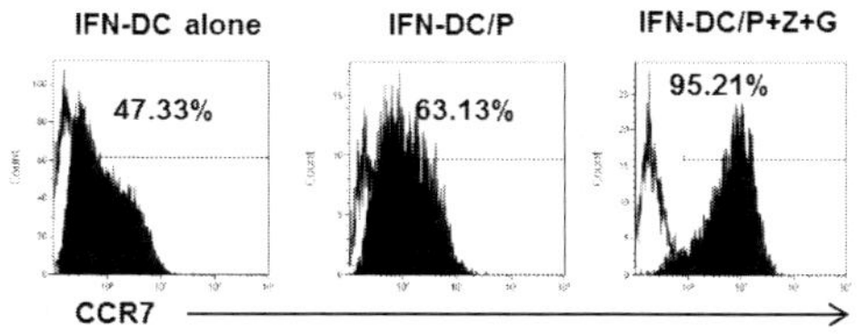

Fig. 2b

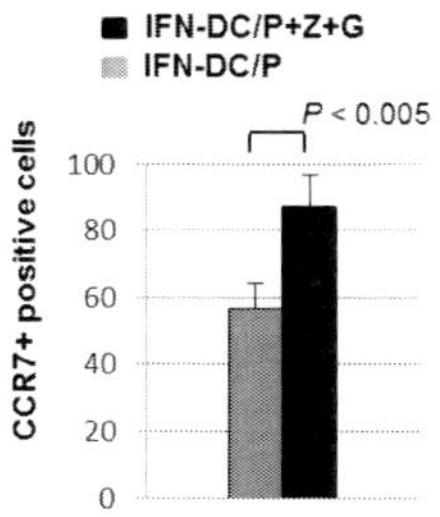

Figure 2. (a) The expression level of CCR7 on IFN-DCs from Pt3 gradually increased following the addition of CMVpp65-peptide alone and the addition of CMVpp65-peptide with zoledronate (Z) plus α-GalCer (G) (b) Statistical analysis of data from four patients with GBM showed that the percentage of CCR7-positive cells among IFN-DCs in the presence of the CMVpp65-peptide with Z plus G was significantly higher than that among IFN-DCs in the presence of the peptide alone.

The cytotoxic activity of expanded cytotoxic T lymphocytes correlates with the frequency of melanoma tetramer-binding CD8+ T cells [4, 23]. To verify our own pentamer results, we assessed the antigen-specific cytotoxic activity of expanding lymphocytes following stimulation "once" by IFN-DCs derived from Pt1 in the presence of the HLA-A*0201-restricted CMVpp65-peptide, Z, and G. Among the expanding lymphocytes, 51.44% were HLA-A*0201-restricted CMVpp65-specific CD8+T cells, 12.12% Vγ9γδT cells, and 0.35% iNKT cells, as shown in Table 2 and Figure 3a-1. As target cells, T98G GBM tumor cell line was used. The results indicate that the effector cells including multifunctional T cells such as antigen-specific CD8+ T cells, Vγ9γδT cells, and iNKT cells efficiently killed T98G tumor cell line in a dose-dependent manner (Figure 3a-2). This dose-dependent lytic activity was very similar to that of expanding lymphocytes following stimulation "twice" by IFN-DCs from Pt1 in the presence of the HLA-A*0201-restricted CMVpp65-peptide alone (Figure 3b-2). Among the expanding lymphocytes, 79.45% were HLA-A*0201-restricted CMVpp65-specific CD8+T cells, 0.57% Vγ9γδT cells, and 0.01% iNKT cells; these were used as effector cells, as shown in Figure 3b-1and Figure 3b-2. The results shown in Figure 3b-1 indicate that T98G cell line expresses the CMVpp65-antigen because effector T cells mainly include CMVpp65-specific CD8+ T cells. Among T98G cell line, 11.5% express PDL1, 3.3% express PDL2 and 100% express MHC-class I (Figure 3C). Blocking experiments using anti-PDL1 and/or anti-PDL2mAb showed that the cytotoxicity of effector cells against T98G cell line did not increase so far as tested (data not shown).

Table 1. Percentage of each population among lymphocytes following stimulation by IFN-DCs in the presence of HLA-A*0101-restricted peptide in different conditions (Pt1)

	CMVpp65-specific CD8+T	γδT	iNKT
Before culture	0.17	1.71	0.06
After culture			
P alone	6.52	0.32	0.00
P + Z	9.06	31.18	0.00
P + G	5.92	2.01	3.49
P + Z + G	10.70	38.05	3.50

Note that the total number of lymphocytes expanded by IFN-DCs in the presence of the CMVpp65-peptide with Z plus G was the highest among the other three different conditions mentioned above for both cases of using the HLA-A*0201-restricted peptide and HLA-A*0101-restricted CMVpp65-peptide (Table 3). Moreover, the total number of CMVpp65-specific CD8+ cells induced by IFN-DCs from two Pts and two HDs who possess HLA-A*0201, in the presence of the HLA-A*0201-restricted CMVpp65-peptide with Z plus G was higher than that in the presence of the peptide alone (Figure 4). The induction ability of CMVpp65-specific CD8+ T cells by IFN-DCs from Pt3 possessing HLA*0101, in the presence of the HLA-A*0101-restricted peptide was similar to that from Pt. 1 (data not shown).

Table 2. Percentage of each population among lymphocytes following stimulation by IFN-DCs in the presence of HLA-A*0201-restricted peptide in different conditions (Pt1)

	CMVpp65-specific CD8+T	γδT	iNKT
Before culture	0.62	1.71	0.06
After culture			
P alone	39.46	0.10	0.01
P + Z	34.83	13.83	0.00
P + G	48.14	0.17	0.48
P + Z + G	51.44	12.12	0.35

Table 3. Total number of lymphocytes following culture for 10 days with autologous IFN-DCs in the presence of the CMVpp65-peptide (HLA-A*0101-restricted or HLA-A*0201-restricted) in different conditions (Pt1)

	HLA-A*0101-restricted peptide	HLA-A*0201-restricted peptide
Before culture	2.0×10^6	2.0×10^6
After culture		
P alone	6.8×10^6	14.0×10^6
P + Z	9.8×10^6	11.2×10^6
P + G	6.8×10^6	10.9×10^6
P + Z + G	11.5×10^6	14.1×10^6

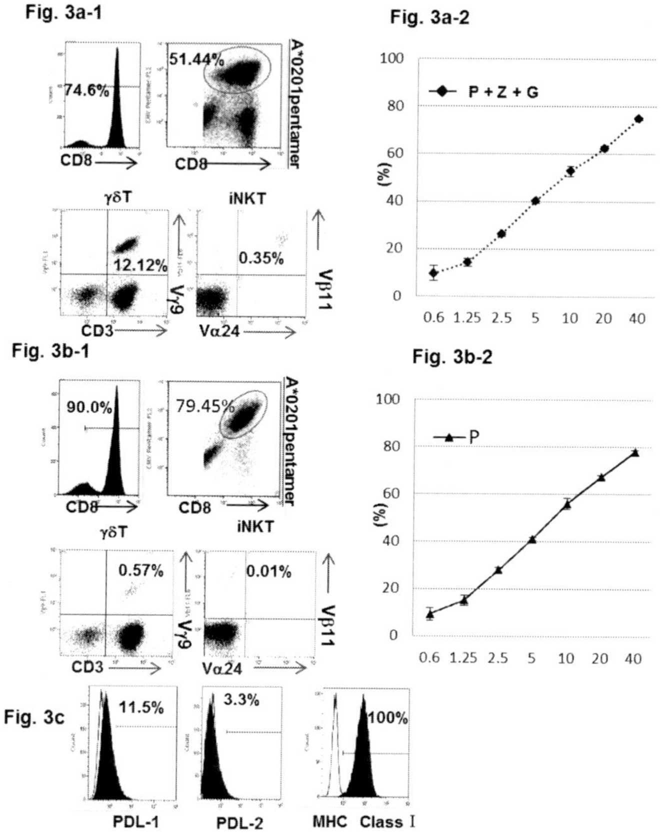

Figure 3. The cytotoxic activity of the expanded lymphocytes including multifunctional T cells such as HLA-A*0201-restricted CMVpp65-specific CD8+ T cells, Vγ9γδT cells, and iNKT cells against the GBM tumor cell line, T98G, is similar to that of the expanded lymphocytes mainly including HLA-A*0201-restricted CMVpp65-specific CD8+ T cells. 3a-1; Phonotypical analysis of the expanding lymphocytes following stimulation "once" by IFN-DCs from Pt1 in the presence of HLA-A*0201-restricted CMVpp65-peptide (P), Z, and G, which were used as effector cells including antigen-specific CD8+ T cells, Vγ9γδT cells, and iNKT cells for the assessment of cytotocix activity against T98G glioblastoma tumor cell line. 3a-2; The cytotoxic activity of the effector cells described in 3a-1, efficiently killed T98G glioblastoma tumor cell line in a dose-dependent manner.
3b-1; Phonotypical analysis of the expanding lymphocytes following stimulation "twice" by IFN-DCs from Pt1 in the presence of HLA-A0201-restricted CMVpp65-peptide (P) alone which were used as effector cells for assessment of cytotocix activity against T98G glioblastoma tumor cell line. 3b-2; The cytotoxic activity of the expanded lymphocytes mainly including HLA-A0201-restricted CMVpp65-specific CD8+ T cells described in 3b-1, efficiently killed T98G in a dose-dependent manner.
(c), Phenotypical analysis of PDL1, PDL2, and MHC class I on T98G glioblastoma tumor cell line used as target cells.

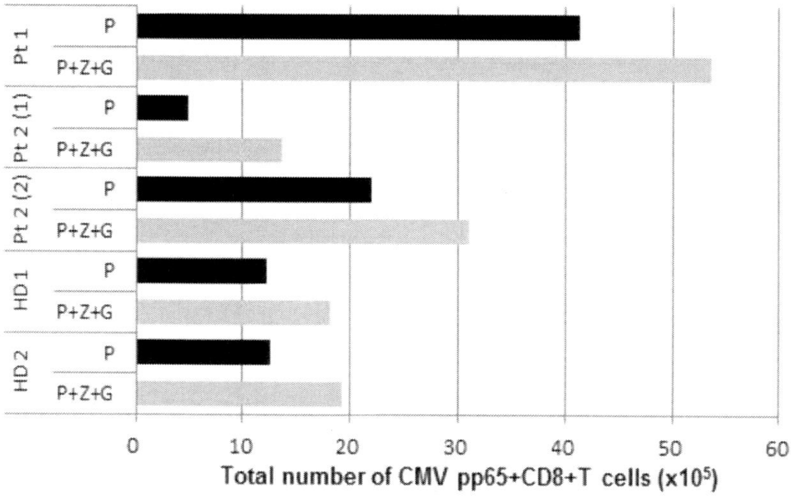

Figure 4. The total number of CMVpp65+CD8+ T cells following 10day-culture of lymphocytes with IFN-DCs in the presence of the HLA-A*0201-restricted CMVpp65-peptide (P), Z, and G was larger than that following culture of lymphocytes with IFN-DCs in the presence of the peptide alone. Pt1, Pt2, HD1, and HD2 are HLA-A*0201-positive. The data for Pt2 (1) and Pt2 (2) were results from PBMCs before DC therapy and from PBMC after seven DC therapies (intervals of 2 weeks, 5 x $10^6$of DCs/infusion) using IFN-DCs pulsed with tumor-lysates, Z, and G., respectively.

It is important to note the case of Pt2 shown in Figures 4 and 5a. In the experiments, the PBMCs were harvested from the first apheresis [Pt2 (1)] (before DC therapy) and compared with PBMCs harvested from the second apheresis [Pt2 (2)] on day 30 following seven DC therapies (intervals of 2 weeks, 5 x 10^6/ infusion) using DCs pulsed with tumor-lysates plus Z and G. The percentage of CD8+ T cells among lymphocytes increased from 29.24% (before DC therapy) to 41.52% (after DC therapy) and the percentage of CMVpp65-specific CD8+ T cells among CD8+T cells increased from 0.08% (before treatment) to 0.20% (after treatment). In this case, it is observed that the percentage of Vγ9γδT cells among lymphocytes also increased from 1.79% (before DC therapy) to 4.54% (on day 30 after DC therapies) (Figure 5a). On the other hand, no increase in the percentage of iNKT cells among lymphocytes on day 30 after DC therapies was observed, presumably owing to the low percentage (0.01%) of iNKT cells among lymphocytes before DC therapy. Furthermore, in an in vitro expansion study using IFN-DCs from the first apheresis (Aphe) product compared with IFN-DCs from the second Aphe product (Figure 5b), the percentage of CMVpp65-specific CD8+ T cells among CD8+T cells expanded by IFN-DCs in the presence of the CMVpp65-peptide alone increased from 22.34% for the first Aphe product to 54.08% for the second Aphe product. In the case of IFN-DCs in the presence of the CMVpp65-peptide, Z, and G, it also increased from 40.37% for the first Aphe product to 58.70% for the second Aphe product. Consequently, the total number of CMVpp65+CD8+T cells following the culture of lymphocytes with autologous IFN-DCs derived from the second apheresis was larger than that from the first apheresis product for the CMVpp65-peptide alone and for the peptide with Z plus G [Pt2 (1) vs Pt2 (2)], as shown in Figure 4.

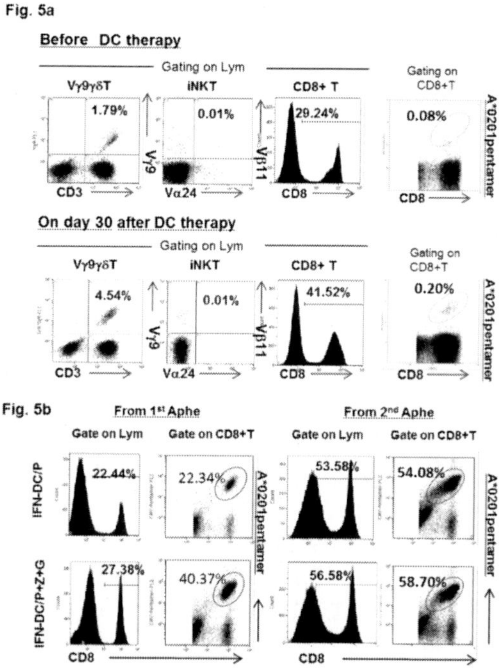

Figure 5. (a) On day 30 following DC therapy using IFN-DCs pulsed with tumor lysates, Z, and G for Pt. 2, the percentages of CD8+ T cells, Vγ9γδT cells, and iNKT cells among lymphocytes (Lym) were shown. The percentages of CD8+ T cells and Vγ9γδT cells among Lym and those of CMVpp-65-specific CD8+ T cells among CD8+ T cells increased.

(b) The percentage of CMVpp65-specific CD8+T cells among CD8+ T cells expanded by IFN-DCs derived from PBMCs after DC therapy was higher than that expanded by IFN-DCs derived from PBMCs before DC therapy under both conditions (with IFN-DCs in the presence of the CMVpp65-peptide alone and IFN-DCs in the presence of the peptide plus Z and G).

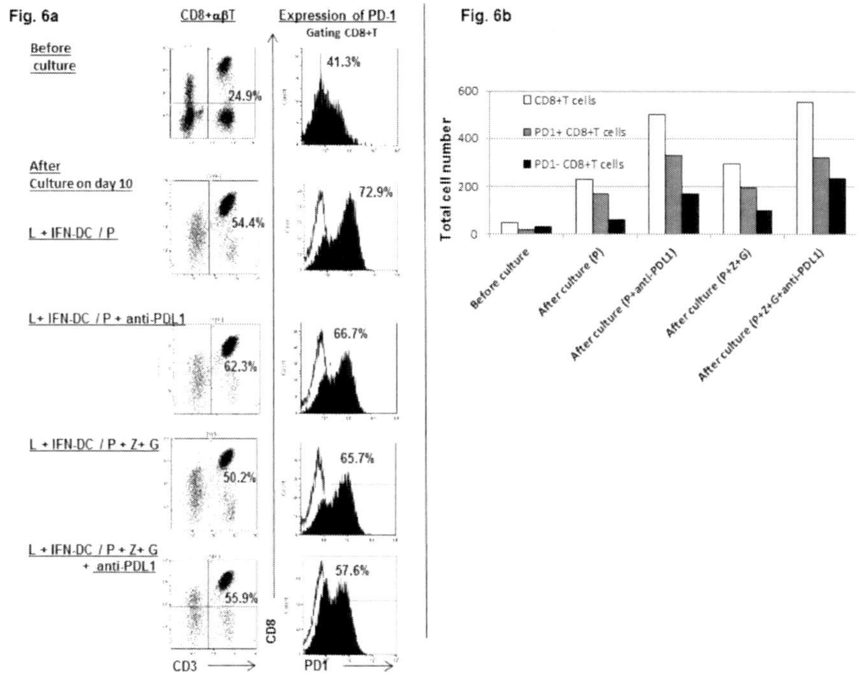

Figure 6. (a) The expression level of PD-1 on CD8+ T cells expanded by IFN-DCs derived from Pt1 in the presence of the CMVpp65-peptide, Z, and G was lower than those on the IFN-DCs pulsed with the peptide alone. In the presence of anti-PDL1mAb, the expression level of PD-1 on CD8+T cells expanded by IFN-DCs decreased under both conditions, in the presence of the CMV-peptide alone or in the presence of the peptide, Z plus G. The expression level of PD-1 on CD8+ T cells following the culture of lymphocytes (L) with IFN-DCs in the presence of the CMVpp65-peptide and Z plus G, and anti-PDL1mAb was lower than that in the presence of the peptide and anti-PDL1mAb (57.6% vs 66.7%).

(b) Among different conditions, a combination of IFN-DCs in the presence of the CMVpp65-peptide, Z, G, and anti-PDL1mAb mostly induced a large number of PD-1-negative CD8+ T cells.

In another experiment, the expression levels of CTLA-4 and PD-1 on CD8+T cells expanded by IFN-DCs from three patients with GBM in the presence of the CMVpp65-peptide, Z, and G were assessed. The results showed that the expression level of CTLA4 was very low whereas the expression level of PD-1 was very high (data not shown). Thus, we focused on the contribution of PDL1 expression on IFN-DCs to the expansion of antigen-specific CD8+ T cells expressing PD-1. Firstly, we assessed the expression levels of PD-1 on CD8+ T cells expanded by IFN-DCs in the presence of the CMVpp65-peptide alone in comparison with that on the cells expanded by IFN-DCs in the presence of the peptide plus Z and G. The results showed that the expression level of PD-1 on CD8+ T cells expanded by IFN-DCs in the presence of the CMVpp65-peptide alone was higher than that on the cells expanded by IFN-DCs in the presence of the peptide plus Z and G (72.9% vs 65.7%) (Figure 6a). Furthermore, when PDL1 expression on IFN-DCs was blocked with anti-PDL1mAb, the expression level of PD-1 on CD8+ T cells was 66.7% for IFN-DCs in the presence of the peptide alone and that of PD-1 on CD8+ T cells was 57.6% for IFN-DCs in the presence of the peptide with Z plus G (Figure 6a). These results indicate that among different conditions, IFN-DCs in the presence of the CMVpp65-peptide, Z, G, and anti-PDL1 mAb mostly induced a large number of PD-1-negative CD8+ T cells. In summary, as shown in Figure 6b, the total number of PD1-negative CD8+T cells was largest in the presence of anti-PDL1mAb in the case of using IFN-DCs in the presence of the CMVpp65-peptide with Z plus G. The results of the experiments for two other patients were similar to those for Pt1 (data not shown).

Cytokine Production in the Supernatant of Co-Culture of Lymphocytes and Autologous IFN-DCs in the Presence of CMVpp65-Peptide, Z, and G

We next examined the production of the cytokines, IFNγ, TNFα, TGFβ, IL-1β, IL-12p70, IL-18, and IL-6 in the supernatant of co-culture of lymphocytes with IFN-DCs in the presence of the CMVpp65-peptide with Z plus G and compared it with that in the supernatant in the presence of the peptide alone. As shown in Figure 7, the supernatant of co-culture of lymphocytes with IFN-DCs in the presence of the CMVpp65-peptide with Z plus G showed higher amounts of Th1 cytokines such as IFNγ and TNFα,which are favorable for the induction of cytotoxic T cells [24] and higher amounts of IL-18, which up-regulate DC function [25], Moreover, lower amounts of IL-6, which down-regulate DC function [26], than those in the supernatant of co-culture of lymphocytes with IFN-DCs were detected in the presence of the peptide alone. TGFβ1, a cytokine with complex functions, modulates cell growth and survival, and plays important roles in the immune system [27]. Its production is similar between two different conditions (CMVpp65-peptide alone and the peptide with Z plus G). IL-1β and IL-12p70 productions by IFN-DCs were very low under any conditions.

Fig. 7a

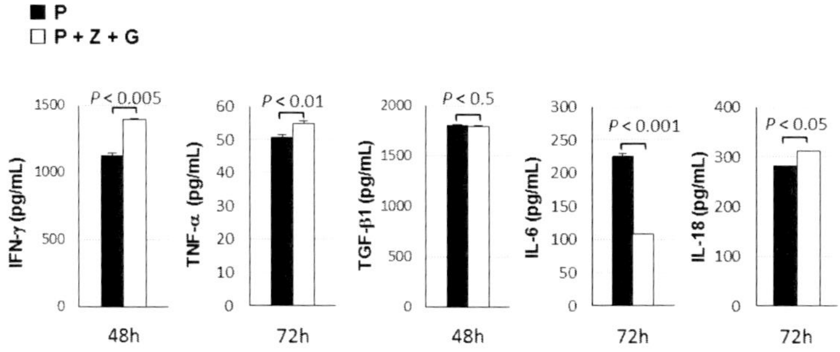

Figure 7. Cytokine production profile in the supernatant following culture of lymphocytes with autologous IFN-DCs in the presence of HLA-A*0201-restricted CMVpp65-peptide alone vs the peptide with Z plus G.

IFNγ, TNFα, IL-1β, IL-12p70, IL-18, TGFβ, and IL-6 secretion amounts were determined by ELISA. Results are represented as the mean±SD of four independent experiments. In the supernatant following culture of IFN-DCs with autologous lymphocytes in the presence of the CMVpp65-peptide with Z plus G, the amounts of IFNγ, TNFα, and IL-18 were higher than those in the supernatant following culture of IFN-DCs with autologous lymphocytes in the presence of the peptide alone. The amount of IL-6 in the presence of the CMVpp65-peptide with Z plus G was lower than that in the presence of CMVpp65-peptide alone. The amount of TGFβ was the same under both conditions in the presence of the CMVpp65- peptide alone and in the presence of the peptide with Z plus G.

DISCUSSION

In this study, we demonstrate the potent, adjuvant effects of the combination of Z and G on tumor-antigen-specific CD8+ T cells. This shows that Vγ9γδT cells activated by Z and iNKT cells activated by G are pivotal in the adjuvant effects, linking innate and adaptive immunities in a way that amplifies the activation and proliferation of tumor -antigen-specific CD8+ T cells. This has a number of important implications, some of which have a significant impact on the use of a combination of Z and G in the setting of cancer therapy.

Accumulating evidence indicates human CMV as a factor contributing to glioma progression [28, 29], and CMV has been suggested as a therapeutic target [30]. Although not classified as an oncogenic virus, CMV can enhance cellular proliferation, angiogenesis, and immune evasion, thus enabling several hallmarks of cancer [31, 32]. More importantly, CMV antigens and nucleic acids have been detected in histological sections of GBM but not in surrounding healthy tissues [33, 34]. Vaccination of one patient with DCs pulsed with autologous GBM lysate elicited a CMV-specific immune response, further supporting the presence of CMV antigens in GBM tissues [7]. These previous observations led us to target CMV antigens with immune-based therapies including DC therapies.

Among many different DC preparation methods in vitro for DC therapy, the use of IFN-DCs in this study had some advantages. It has been reported that CD56+ γδT cells are potent antitumor effectors more capable of killing tumor cells than CD56- γδT cells [24]. Furthermore, cytolytic effector function of circulating human CD8+ T cells closely correlate with CD56 expression, in which a marked oligoclonal expansion is confined to the CD56+ subset of CD8+ T cells [35]. Moreover, compared with the most commonly used DC populations, namely mature IL-4DCs, IFN-DCs expressing CD56 predominantly expand CD56+ A27L-specific CD8+T cells and CD56+ Vγ9γδT cells in the presence of the Mart-1-modified A27L antigen and Z [13]. Considering these previous observations, we used IFN-DCs in this study and discovered that using them has several advantages as follows.

The chemokine-receptor protein CCR7 is a key factor for the efficient migration of activated DCs to lymph nodes where they interact with T cells [8]. Notably, the expression level of CCR7 on IFN-DCs is significantly much higher than that on mIL-4 DCs, and expression level of CCR7 on IFN-DCs gradually increased after incubation with the CMVpp65-peptide with Z plus G (Figures 2a and 2b). This indicates that IFN-DCs pulsed with the peptide, Z, and G have high trafficking activity across endothelial cells to lymph nodes where they interact with antigen-specific CD8+T cells.

PD-1, an immunoreceptor belonging to the CD28/CTLA-4 family, negatively regulates the antigen receptor interacting with either of two ligands, PDL1 or PDL2 [20]. Accumulating evidence shows the promising future for the clinical applications of PD-1 agonists and antagonists to various human diseases including autoimmunity, tumor immunity, infectious immunity, transplantation immunity, allergy, and immunological privilege. The PD-1/PDL1 pathway is an important element contributing to tumor-mediated immune suppression [20, 36, 37]. Ligation of PD-1 results in T cell inactivation and apoptosis and plays a key role in modulating the delicate balance between tolerance and immune activation. The inappropriate upregulation of PD-1 expression by T cells has been shown to promote an exhausted phenotype facilitating the development of chronic viral infection [18]. In contrast, PD-1 blockade results in the restoration of functionally active T cells and clearance of infection. The PD-1/PDL1 pathway is also being evaluated as a central mechanism by which tumors escape host immunity. The expression of PDL1 on tumor has been demonstrated in several tumor models and is considered to play a significant role in promoting tolerance by binding PD-1 on activated T cells. In addition, the expression of PDL1 on tumor cells has been shown to directly inhibit T-cell-mediated lysis owing to the inactivation of tumor-reactive cytotoxic T lymphocytes. It has been demonstrated that tumor cells such as myeloma cells and DC/tumor fusions highly express PDL1 wherein PDL1 blockade was associated with enhanced cytotoxic T-lymphocyte-mediated killing of myeloma cells [37].

In our previous study of healthy donors and melanoma patients [13], we showed that the induction ability of A27L-specific CD8+ T cells by IFN-DCs was higher than that by mIL-4DCs. In this study, the expression levels of PDL1 and PDL2 on IFN-DCs were significantly lower than those on mIL-4DCs (Figure 1a). Taken together with these observations, we speculate that the higher induction ability of A27L-specific CD8+ T cells by IFN-DCs pulsed with the A27L peptide may partly be due to the lower expression level of PDL1 on IFN-DCs than on mIL-4DCs.

Administration of anti-PDL1 mAb to cancer patients is shown in eradicating tumors in some cancer patients [38-41] In this study, we observed that the expression level of PD-1 on CD8+ T cells expanded by IFN-DCs in the presence of the CMVpp65-peptide, Z, and G was lower than that expanded by IFN-DCs in the presence of the peptide alone (65.7% vs 72.9%) (Figure 6a). In addition, blocking experiments using anti-PDL1mAb showed that among different conditions, using IFN-DCs in the presence of the CMVpp65-peptide, Z, and G together with anti-PDL1mAb, the expression level of PD-1 on CD8+ T cells is the lowest (57.6%) (Figure 6a), which resulted in the largest induction of PD-1 negative CD8+ T cells (Figure 6b), which may be associated with the effective killing of tumors expressing PDL1. These results suggest that anti-PDL1mAb administration together with DC therapy using IFN-DCs pulsed with the CMVpp65-peptide with Z plus G in patients with GBM may enhance antitumor immune responses.

In this study, the cytotoxicity of effector T cells containing CMV-pp65-specific CD8+ T cells efficiently killed T98G tumor cell line in a dose-dependent manner (Figures 3a-2 and 3b-2). However, the killing was not enhanced in the presence of anti-PDL1 and/or anti-PDL2mAb, presumably owing to the low expression levels of on PDL1 and PDL2 on T98G cell line (Figure 3c). We need to further investigate whether the administration of anti-PDL1 and/or anti-PDL2mAb is effective for patients with glioblastoma.

Memory CD8+ T cells are a principal component of immunity against intracellular pathogens such as viruses and they are distinguished by their capacities to survive in the long term, undergo rapid and robust proliferation, and acquire effector function upon antigen re-exposure [42]. In this study, it is important to note that the increase in the percentages of antigen-specific CD8+T cells and Vγ9γδT cells among lymphocytes remained on day 30 after the last administration of IFN-DCs pulsed with tumor lysate, Z, and G in Pt2 with GBM (Figure 5a). In the vitro expansion study (Figure 5b), a more robust expansion of CMVpp65-specific CD8+ T cells was observed using IFN-DCs from the second apheresis product than using IFN-DCs from the first apheresis product, in the presence of the CMVpp65-peptide alone and in the presence of the peptide with Z plus G. These results suggest that following multiple administrations of DCs pulsed with tumor lysates from a patient, some of the tumor antigen-specific CD8+ T cells remained as memory CD8+ T cells in peripheral blood.

Th1 cytokines such as IFNγ and TNFα increase antitumor activity by inhibiting tumor growth and activating components of adoptive immune systems [24]. TGFβ1 has been shown to inhibit the differentiation of CD4+ T cells into Th1 effectors [27]. In this study, the productions of Th1 cytokines such as IFNγ and TNFα by IFN-DCs in the presence of the CMVpp65-peptide with Z plus G were higher than that by IFN-DCs in the presence of the peptide alone. However, TGFβ 1 production by IFN-DCs in the presence of the peptide with Z plus G was lower than that by IFN-DCs in the presence of the peptide alone. These results suggest that the adjuvant effects of Z and G are associated with production of favorable cytokine for anticancer immune responses.

DCs produce a wide range of cytokines depending on their maturation stage, including IL-1, IL-5, TNF-α, IL-12, and IL-23 [43]. IFN-DCs secrete large amounts of inflammatory cytokines such as IL-1β, IL-6, IL-10, IL-18, and TNFα and induction/expression of IL-12 seems restricted to maturing DCs [25]. In this study, IL-12p70 was not detected under any condition, indicating that IFN-DCs are semimature DCs even after pulsing the tumor peptide, Z, and G, as reflected by the higher expression levels of CD36 molecules on IFN-DCs than on mIL-4DCs, as shown in Figure 1a and 1b. The reported biological activities of IL-18 include stimulation of activated T cell proliferation, NK cell activation, and inductions of IFNγ and GM-CSF by activated T lymphocytes and macrophages [25]. IL-6 participates in immunoregulation and inflammatory reaction and there is evidence showing that IL-6 expressed in the glioma may promote glioma growth [44]. Furthermore, a recent study showed that IL-6 down-regulates HLA class II expression and IL-12 production of DCs, which impair the activation of antigen-specific CD4+ T cells [26]. In this study, amount of IL-18 produced was higher when using IFN-DCs in the presence of the CMVpp65-peptide, Z, and G, than when using the peptide alone. Moreover, the amount of IL-6 produced was lower when using IFN-DCs in the presence of the CMVpp65-peptide, Z, and G, than when using the peptide alone (Figure 7). These results also indicate the favorable adjuvant effect of Z and G in terms of the enhancement of tumor antigen-specific CD8+ cell induction.

The adjuvant effect by a combination of Z-activated Vγ9γδT cells with G-activated iNKT cells on antigen-specific CD8+ T cells were similar when stimulator DCs were washed to remove extracellular tumor antigens, Z, and G, as when pulsed DCs and lymphocytes were cocultured in the presence of the additional tumor antigens, Z, and G. These observations support the possibility that our in vitro observations could be translated into the clinical applicatins if DCs pulsed with the tumor antigen, Z, and G are administered therapeutically.

The observed favorable in vitro expansion of CMVpp65-specific CD8+ T cells in response to DCs in the presence of added IL-2 indicates that additional, exogenous IL-2 may also be required to maximize the immunotherapeutic benefits of DCs pulsed with a tumor antigen, Z, and G in clinical settings. It has been shown recently that like DCs, γδT cells present antigens to αβ T cells [45, 46]. It is conceivable that γδT cells, activated in vivo, for example, by administered DCs pulsed with tumor antigen, Z and G, might play a role as APCs, where they can up-take apoptotic bodies from tumor cells and subsequently induce tumor antigen-specific CD8+ T cells in vivo wherein iNKT cell may function as helper T cells producing large amounts of IFNγ. This is indicted by the observation that, following the administration of α-GalCer-pulsed DCs, iNKT cells are expanded as shown by our previous in vivo study [6]. It is important notice that the helper function of a combination of Vγ9γδT and iNKT cells is not MHC-unrestricted, suggesting that the adjuvants effect of a combination of Z and G is theoretically available for all cancer patients.

In summary, this is the first time to demonstrate the adjuvants effect of Z and G on the induction of antigen-specific CD8+ T cells using IFN-DCs. This effect may be a physiologically and therapeutically important bridge between innate and adaptive immunities through DCs. Our findings are anticipated to facilitate the design of more effective immune therapy strategies for patients with malignancies and may provide important insights into immune responses to infectious agents.

REFERENCES

[1] Raval, R. R., Sharabi, A. B., Walker, A. J., Drake, C. G. and Sharma, P. P. (2014). Tumor immunology and cancer immunotherapy: summary of the 2013 SITC primer. *Journal for Immunotherapy of Cancer*. 2,14-24.

[2] Pyzer, A. R., Avigan, D. E. and Rosenblatt, J. (2014). Clinical trials of dendritic cell-based cancer vaccines in hematologic malignancies *Human Vaccines & Immunotherapeutics* 10, 3125-3131.

[3] Castella, B., Riganti, C., Fiore, F., Pantaleoni, F., Canepari, M. E., Peola, S., Foglietta, M., Palumbo, A., Bosia, A., Marta Coscia, M., Boccadoro, M. and Massaia, M. (2011). Immune modulation by zoledronic acid in human myeloma: An advantageous cross-talk between Vγ9VδT cells, αβ CD8+ T cells, Regulatory T cells, and Dendritic cells. *J. Immunol;* 187,1578-1590.

[4] Takahara, M., Miyai, M., Tomiyama, M., Mutou, M., Andrew, J. N. and Nieda, M. (2008). Copulsing tumor antigen-pulsed dendritic cells with zoledronate efficiently enhance the expansion of tumor antigen-specific CD8+ T cells via Vγ9γδT cell activation. *Journal of Leukocyte Biology*. 83,742-754.

[5] Dhodapkar, M.V. and Richter, J. (2011). Harnessing Natural Killer T (NKT) cells in Human Myeloma: Progress and Challenges. *Clin Immunol*. 140:160-166.

[6] Nieda, M., Okai, M., Tazbirkova, A., Lin, H., Yamaura, A., Ide, K., Abraham, R., Juji, T., Mcfariane, D.J. and Nicol, A.J. (2004). Therapuetic activation of Vα24+Vβ11+NKT cells in human subjects results in highly coordinated secondary activation of acquired and innate immunity. *Blood*. 103, 383-389.

[7] Prins, R.M., Cloughesy, T.F., and Linda, M. and Liau, L.M. (2008). Induction of Cytomegrovirus-specific Anti-tumor Immunity after autologus tumor lysate-pulsed dendritic cell vaccination in a patient with glioblastoma. *N Eng J Med.* 359, 539-541.

[8] Sabado, R.L. and Bhardwaj, N. (2015). Dendritic-cell vaccines on the move. *Nature* 519, 300-301.

[9] Nair, S. K., Leon, G. D., Boczkowski, D., Schimitting, R., Xie, W., Staats, J., Liu, R., Jonson, L.A., Weinhold, K., Archer, G.E., Sampson, J. H. and Mitchell, D.A. (2014). Recognition and Killing of Autologus, Primary Glioblastoma Tumor Cellss by Human Cytomegalovirus pp65-Specific Cytotoxic T cells. *Clin Cancer Res.* 20, 2684-2694.

[10] Schuessler, A., Smith, C., Beegley, L., Boyle, G. M., Rehan, S., Matthews, K., Jones, L., Crough, T., Dasari, V., Klein, K., Smalley, A., Alexander, H., Walker, D. G. and Khanna, R. (2014). Auotlogous T-cell therapy for Cytomegraovirus as a Consolidative Treatment for Recurrent Glioblastoma. *Cancer Res.* 74, 3466-3476.

[11] Imperato J.P., Paleologos N.A. and Vick, NA (1990). Effects of treatment on long-term survivors with malignant astrocytomas. *Ann Neurol.* 28, 818-22.

[12] Stupp, R., Mason, W.P., van den Bent, M.J., Weller, M., Fisher, B., Taphoom, M. J. B., Belanger, K., Brandes, A. A., Marosi, C., Bogdahn, U., Curschmann, J., Janzer, R.C., Ludwin S. K., Gorlia, T., Allgeier, A., Lacombe, D., Cairncross, J. G., Eisenhauer, E. and Mirimanoff, R. O. (2005). Radiotherapy plus concomitant and adjuvant temozolomide for glioblastoma. *N Eng J Med.* 352, 987-996.

[13] Nieda, M., Terunuma, H., Eiraku, Y., Deng, X. and Nicol, A.J. (2015). Effective induction of melanoma-antigen-specific CD8+ T cells via Vγ9γδT cell expansion by CD56high+ Interferon-α-induced dendritic cells. *Exp Dermatol.* 24, 35-41.

[14] Carreno, B.M. and Collins, M. (2000). The B7 family of ligands and its receptor: new pathways for costimulation and inhibition of immune responses. *Annu Rev Immunol* 20, 29-53.

[15] Carreno, B.M. and Collins, M. (2003). BTLA:a new inhibitory receptor with a B7-like ligand. *Trends Immunol.* 24, 524-527.

[16] Yamazaki, T., Akiba, H., Iwai, H., Matusda, H., Aoki, M., Tanno, Y., Shin, T., Tsuchiya, H., Pardol, D.M., Okumura, K., Azuma, M. and Yagita, H. (2002). Expression of programmed death 1 ligands by murine T cells and APC. *J. Immunol.* 169, 5538-5545.

[17] Mueller, S.N. and Mackay, L.K. (2016). Tissue-resident memory T cells: local specialities in immune defence. *Nature Reviews Immunology* 16, 79-89.

[18] Blank, C. and Mackensen, A. (2007). Contribution of the PD-L1/PD-1 pathway to T-cell exhaustion: an update on implications for chronic infections and tumor evasion. *Cancer Immunol Immunother* 56, 739-745.

[19] Pardoll, D.M. (2012). The blockade of immune checkpoints in cancer immunotherapy. *Nature Reviews Cancer.* 12, 252-263.

[20] Okazaki, T. and Honjo, T. (2007). PD-1 and PD-1 ligands: from discovery to clinical application. *Internaitonal Immunology* 19, 813-824.

[21] Ueda, R., Ohkusu-Tsukada, K., Fusaki, N., Soeda, A., Kawase, T., Kawakami, Y. and Toda, M. (2010). Identification of HLA-A2- and 24-restricted T cell epitopes derived from SOX6 expressed in glioma stem cells for immunotherapy; *Int. J, Cancer,* 126, 919-929.

[22] Sasawatari, S., Tadaki, T., Isogai, M., Takahara, M., Nieda, M. and Kakimi, K. (2006). Efficient priming and expansion of antigen-specific CD8+ T cells by a novel cell-based artificial APC. *Immunol. Cell Biol,* 84, 512-521.

[23] Paczesny, S., Banchereau, J., Wittkowski, K. M., Saracino, G., Fay, J. and Palucka A. K. (2004). Expression of melanoma-specific cytotoxic CD8+ T cell precursors in patient with metastatic melanoma vaccinated with CD34+ progenitor-derived dendritic cells. *J. Exp. Med.* 199, 1503-1511.

[24] Gruenbacher, G., Gander, H., Rahm, A., Nussbaumer, W., Romani, N. and Thurnher, M. (2009). CD56+ human blood dendritic cells effectively promote Th1-type γδT cells responses. *Blood.* 114,4422-4431.

[25] Mohty, M., Vialle-Castellano, A., Nunes, J.A., Isnardon, D., Olive, D. and Gaugler, B. (2003). IFN-α skews monocyte differentiation into Toll-like receptor 7-expressing dendritic cells with potent functional activities. *J Immunol.* 171, 3385-93.

[26] Ohno, Y., Kitamura, H., Takahashi, N., Ohtake, J., Kaneumi, S., Sumida, K., Homma, S., Kawamura, H., Minagawa, N., Shibasaki, S. and Taketomi, A. (2016). IL-6 down-regulates HLA class Ⅱ expression and IL-12 production of human dendritic cells to impair activation of antigen-specific CD4(+) T cells. *Cancer Immunol Immunother,* 65,193-204.

[27] Dumitriu, I. E., Dunber, D. R., Howie, S. E., Sethi, T. and Gregory, C.D. (2009). Human dendritic cells produce TGF-β1 under the influence of Lung Carcinoma Cells and Prime the differentiation of CD4+CD25+FoxP3 regulatory T cells. *Immunology,* 182, 2295-2807.

[28] Cinatl, J., Scholz, M., Kotchetkov, R., Vogel, J.U. and Doerr, H.W. (2004). Molecular mechanisms of the modulatory effects of HCMV infection in tumor cell biology. *Trends Mol Med*, 10, 19-23.

[29] Michaelis, M., Baumgarten, P., Mittelbronn, M., Driever, P.H., Doerr, H.W. and Cinatl, J. Jr. (2011). Oncomodulation by human cytomegraovirus: novel clinical findings open new reads. *Med Microbiol Immunol.* 200,1-5.

[30] Johnsen, J.I., Baryawno, N. and Soederberg-Naucler, C. (2011). Is human cytomegalovirus a target in cancer therapy? *Oncotarget* 2, 1329-1338.

[31] Soroceanu, L. and Cobbs, C.S. (2011). Is HCMV a tumor promoter? *Virus Res* 157, 193-203.

[32] Dziurzynski, K., Chang, S.M., Heimberger, A.B., Kalejta, R.F., McGregor Dallas S.R., Smit, M., Soroceanu, L. and Cobbs, C.S. (2012). HCMV and Glioma Symposium. Consensus on the role of human cytomegalovirus in glioblastoma. *Neuro Oncol.* 14, 246-255.

[33] Cobbs, C.S., Harkins, L., Samanta, M., Gillespie, G.Y., Bharara, S., King, P.H., Nabors, L.B., Cobbs, C.G. and Britt, W.J. (2002). Human cytomegarovirous infeiton and expression in human malignant glioma. *Cancer Res.* 62, 3347-3350.

[34] Ghazi, A., Ashoori, A., Hanley, P.J., Brawley, V.S., Shaffer, D.R., Kew, Y., Powell, S.Z., Grossman, R., Grada, Z., Scheurer, M.E., Hegde, M., Leen, A.M., Bollard, C.M., Rooney, C.M., Heslop, H.E., Gottschalk, S. and Ahmed, N. (2012). Generation of polylonal CMV-specific T cells for the adoptive immunotherapy of glioblasotma. *J Immunother.* 35,159-168.

[35] Pittet, M. J., Speiser, D.E., Valmori, D., Cerottini, J.C. and Romero, P. (2006). Cutting edge: cytolytic effector function in human circulating CD8+ T cells closely correlates with CD56 surface expression. *J. Immunol.* 164,1148-1152.

[36] Berger, R., Rotem-Yehudar, R., Slama, G., Landes, S., Kneller, A., Leiba, M., Koren-Michowitz, M., Shimoni, A. and Nagler, A. (2008). Phase I Safety and Pharmacokinetics Study of CT-011, a Humanized Antibody Intercting with PD-1, in Patients with Advanced Hematologic Malignancies. *Clin Cancer Res* 14, 3044-3051.

[37] Rosenblatt, J., Glozbecker, B., Mills, H., Vasir, B., Tzachanis, D., Levine, J.D., Joyce, R.M., Wellenstein, K., Keefe, W., Schickler, M., Rotem-Yehudar, R., Kufe, D. and Avigan, D. (2011). PD-1 blockade by CT-011, anti PD-1 antibody, enhances ex-vivo T cell responses to autotogous dendritic/ myeloma fusion vaccine. *J. Immunnother.* 34, 409-418.

[38] Berger, R., Rotem-Yehudar, R., Slama, G., Landes, S., Kneller, A., Leiba, M., Kore-Michowitz, M., Shimoni, A. and Naglaer, A. (2008). Phase I Safety and Pharmacokinetic Study of CT-011, a Humanized Antibody Interacting with PD-1, in Paitents with Advanced Hematologic Malignancies. *Clin Cancer Res* 14, 3044-3051.

[39] Pardoll, D.M. (2012). The blockade of immune checkpoints in cancer immunotherapy. *Nature Reviews* 12, 252-264.

[40] Swaika, A., Hammond, W.A. and Joseph, R.W. (2015). Current state of anti-PDL1 and PD-1 agents in cancer therapy, 2015. *Mol Immunol.* 67, 4-17.

[41] Brahmer, J.R., Tykodi, S. S., Chow, L.Q.M., Hwu, W. J., Topalian,S.L., Hwu, P., Drake, C.G., Camacho, L.H., Kauh, J., Odunsi, K., Pitot, H.C., Hamid, O., Bhatia, S., Martins, R., Eaton, K., Chen, S., Salay, T. M., Alaparthy, S., Grosso, J.F., Korman, A.J., Parker, S.M., Agrawal, S., Goldberg, S.M., Pardoll, D.M., Gupta, A. and Wigginton, J. M. (2012). Safety and Activity of Anti-PD-L1 Antibody in Patients with Advanced Cancer. *The New England Journal of Medicine***.** 336, 2455-2465.

[42] Laidlaw, B.J., Craft, J. E. and Kaech, S. M. (2016). The multifaced role of CD4+ T cells in CD8+ T cell memory. *Nature Reviews Immunology.* 16, 102-111.

[43] Collin, M., McGovern, N. and Haniffa, M. (2013). Human dendritic cell subsets. *Immunology,* 140, 22-30.

[44] Shan, Y., He, X., Song, W., Han, D., Niu, J. and Wang, J. (2015). Role of IL-6 in the invasiveness and prognosis of glioma. *Int J Clin Med.* 8, 9114-9120.

[45] Brandes, M., Willimann, K. and Moser, B. (2005). Professional antigen-presentation function by human γδ T cells. *Science,* 309, 264-268.

[46] Muto, M., Baghdadi, M., Maekawa, R., Wada, H. and Seino, K. (2015). Myeloid molecular characterization of human γδT cells support their acquisition of tumor antigen-presenting capacity; *Cancer Immunol Immunother,* 64, 941-949.

In: Horizons in Cancer Research. Volume 63 ISBN: 978-1-53610-013-6
Editor: Hiroto S. Watanabe

Chapter 5

REGULATION OF CD8⁺ T CELLS IN THE SKIN AND IMPLICATIONS FOR THE DEVELOPMENT OF SQUAMOUS CELL CARCINOMA

Jazmina L. Cruz and James W. Wells*
The University of Queensland Diamantina Institute,
Brisbane, Australia

ABSTRACT

The skin is the largest organ in the human body weighing ~3.6 kg and covering ~$2m^2$ in the average adult. It is the first line of defence against external aggressions and acts as a passive barrier against physical traumas and environmental insults. The fact that healthy skin contains more than twice the number of $CD8^+$ T cells found in the blood (approx. $2x10^{10}$ cells), underlines the key role of the skin in protection from infection and carcinogens and emphasizes the importance of this population in the maintenance of skin homeostasis. The crucial anti-tumour role played by T cells in the skin is clearly demonstrated by the high rate of skin tumour formation in organ transplant patients who receive T cell suppressive drugs to maintain the integrity of their

* Corresponding Author address: The University of Queensland Diamantina Institute, The University of Queensland, Translational Research Institute, 37 Kent Street, Brisbane, QLD 4102, Australia. Email: j.wells3@uq.edu.au.

transplanted organs. These patients show a 10-100 fold increased risk of cutaneous squamous cell carcinoma (SCC) development compared to healthy patients, and indeed, some renal transplant patients currently presenting to the Princess Alexandra Hospital, Brisbane, Australia, require the removal of ~120 primary skin tumours each year. However, although this relationship has been well-documented, it is still very unclear which T cell populations or mechanisms mediate cancer protection in the skin. This chapter will address $CD8^+$ T cell activation and regulation in the skin, paying special attention to what it is known about $CD8^+$ T cell activity and its link with SCC development.

Keywords: CD8, T cell, skin, squamous cell carcinoma, regulation

INTRODUCTION

The skin provides an immediate physical barrier between internal tissues and the environment. This essential organ plays a key role in protecting the body against pathogens, preventing excessive water loss, permitting sensation, and regulating body temperature. The skin is also an important site for immune system development, as recently highlighted by the finding that the skin microbiome plays a critical role in the establishment of a healthy immune system [1, 2]. In turn, a perfectly functioning immune system is essential to skin homeostasis, as inappropriate or misdirected immune activity can lead to the breakdown of skin integrity [3]. However, there is a critical knowledge gap in our understanding of how cellular mechanisms contribute to the maintenance of skin homeostasis, and particularly how immune cells, which can become potentially dangerous if dysregulated, are regulated in the skin.

T cells are white blood cells that mature in the Thymus, hence the name "T cell." There are several subsets of T cells, each with a distinct function, and the skin is a major reservoir for these cells [4]. The $CD8^+$ T cell subset plays a critical protective role by recognizing and destroying virally-infected- and malignant cells [5, 6], and influencing other cells through production of cytokines such as interferon (IFN)-γ [7, 8] and tumor necrosis factor (TNF) [9]. In the skin, $CD8^+$ T cells are responsible for immune surveillance and contribute to the prevention of infection. While most self-reactive $CD8^+$ T cells are deleted in the thymus during development through central tolerance mechanisms, this process is incomplete and peripheral tolerance is required to prevent the destruction of host tissues [10-14]. Not surprisingly, the activation of $CD8^+$ T cells is tightly regulated to avoid the unwanted destruction of healthy, normal cells. However, the mechanisms that tightly regulate memory/effector T cell populations in the skin are not well understood, and represent a critical gap in our knowledge.

Multiple immune cell populations, including classical $CD4^+Foxp3^+$ regulatory T cells [15] (T-reg), invariant natural-killer T cells [16, 17] and $CD11b^+Gr\text{-}1^+$ myeloid-derived suppressor cells [18] are implicated in the control of $CD8^+$ T cells in the skin. $CD4^+Foxp3^+$ T-reg are especially abundant in the skin and modulate $CD8^+$ T cell differentiation and effector function *in vivo* by critically regulating IL-2 homeostasis [19]. Experimentally depleting $CD4^+Foxp3^+$ T-reg from the skin leads to increased $CD8^+$ T cell priming and enhanced allergic skin reactions [20]. Production of the immunosuppressive cytokine IL-10 by $CD4^+Foxp3^+$ T-regs resident in lymph nodes has been implicated in the induction of $CD8^+$ T cells that suppress contact hypersensitivity reactions in the skin [21]. Other immune populations with regulatory potential include $CD4^+CD8^+$ double-positive T cells [22, 23], regulatory macrophages, which inhibit T cell proliferation through inducible nitric oxide synthase [24] (iNOS), and plasmacytoid dendritic cells (pDC), which by expression of indoleamine 2,3 dioxygenase [25] (IDO) can reduce the T cell stimulatory potential of dendritic cells (DC). While not yet fully characterized, we have some understanding of how these cellular mechanisms work. However, the potential of other immune populations to regulate $CD8^+$ T cell responses in the skin is poorly explored.

Upon antigen stimulation, naïve T cells rapidly undergo terminal differentiation to effector and memory T cells. Compared to naive T cells, activated and memory T cells are more sensitive to antigen stimulation, exhibit faster response kinetics, reduced dependence on costimulation and can respond to lower affinity ligands. Memory T cells may be more resistant to the induction of apoptosis by virtue of increased expression of anti-apoptotic Bcl-2, although this may vary between central memory (T_{CM}) and effector memory (T_{EM}) T cells [26]. Terminal T cell differentiation transforms antigen-specific T cells from a naïve population, possessing a highly malleable differentiation potential, to committed effector and memory populations which have little or no plasticity and a reduced requirement for costimulation. This has led to the belief that they are resistant to inactivation or tolerance induction [27]. Indeed, memory $CD8^+$ T cells have been shown to provide a potent barrier to transplantation tolerance induction [28].

Recently, a new memory population, known as tissue-resident memory (T_{RM}), has been described that is phenotypically and functionally distinct from T_{CM} and T_{EM} [29, 30]. T_{RM} populations play an important role in protective immunity to site-specific pathogens in the lung and skin [30-32], and unlike other memory populations they do not recirculate [29]. T_{RM} can be clearly distinguished from other memory T cell populations by the expression of the CD103 integrin, which binds to the $\alpha_E\beta_7$ integrin expressed by keratinocytes, and it has been hypothesized that this interaction may help T_{RM} to maintain their location within the skin [33]. Importantly, T_{RM} have now been described in multiple sites other than the skin [34] and understanding how this unique subset of $CD8^+$ T cells is regulated is crucial.

Adaptive Immunity and $CD8^+$ T Cells

The adaptive or acquired immune system is comprised of a set of highly specialized cells, T cells and B cells, which mount antigen-specific responses against foreign pathogens, and establish long-lasting immunological memory designed to trigger a rapid and robust recall response upon antigen re-exposure [35]. The capacity of T cells to recognize specific antigens rests on the tremendous diversity of their T cell receptors (TCR), which recognize cognate peptide bound to major histocompatibility complex molecules (MHC) displayed on the surface of professional antigen presenting cells (APCs) [36]. Naïve cytotoxic $CD8^+$ T cells circulate between the blood and secondary lymphoid organs where they become activated through their interaction with mature APCs. To enter into the lymph nodes naive $CD8^+$ T cells typically express on their cell surface the homing factors CC-chemokine receptor 7 (CCR7), which signaling pathway activates LFA1 (lymphocyte function-associated antigen 1) that binds ICAM1 (intercellular adhesion molecule 1) on the surface of the endothelium, and CD62L (L-selectin) that binds to the high endothelial venules, allowing the blood circulating lymphocytes to directly enter the lymph nodes [37-39]. After cognate antigen recognition, activated antigen specific $CD8^+$ T cells undergo clonal expansion and differentiate into effector T cells (T_E). This phase is known as the "expansion phase" in which a single precursor can experience more than 15 divisions over the course of 1 week [40]. Once activated, the T_E cells down-regulate the expression of CCR7 and CD62L and egress the secondary lymphoid organs to patrol the peripheral tissues and eliminate target cells by releasing cytolytic granules containing granzymes and perforin [41, 42]. This is known as the "effector phase." The production of IL-12 by activated macrophages/monocytes and dendritic cells during microbial infection stimulates the T_E cells to secrete interferon-γ, which links the adaptive immune response with the innate immune response [43]. The release of cytokines/chemokines, such as IL-1, IL-8 and TNF, and the expression of unique combinations of selectin and integrin molecules in the infected and/or inflamed tissues set up an "area code" which favors the recall of antigen-specific T_E cells into the target organ [41]. At the same time and rapidly after priming, T_E cells express tissue-homing factors on their surface. The idea that antigen-experienced T cells have specific tissue-tropism was demonstrated by the fact that adoptively transferred lymphocytes mainly infiltrate the tissues from where they were isolated [44, 45]. For instance, T_E cells primed to migrate to the skin preferentially up-regulate CC-chemokine receptor (CCR)4 and/or CCR10, as well as cutaneous leukocyte antigen (CLA) which is a ligand of both endothelial-cell selectin (E-selectin) and platelet selectin (P-selectin) constitutively expressed by dermal micro vessels [46, 47]. Conversely, T_E cells activated in the gastrointestinal associated lymph nodes up-regulate the $\alpha 4\beta 7$ integrin and CCR9, which bind the mucosal vascular addressin cell-adhesion molecule 1 (MADCAM1) and the CC-chemokine ligand 25 (CCL25) respectively; both of these ligands are expressed by epithelial cells in the small intestine [48-50].

Once the "expansion phase" is concluded, between 90 to 95% of the antigen-specific $CD8^+$ T cells undergo apoptosis. This stage is known as "contraction phase" and is believed to be important to avoid the prevalence of certain T cell clones and preserve the diversity of the T cell repertoire of the organism [51]. However, a small subset of antigen-specific T cells survive the contraction phase giving rise to long-lived "memory" T cells (T_M). T_M ($CD62L^+CCR7^+$) which circulate between blood and secondary lymphoid tissues are known as "central memory" T cells (T_{CM}), whereas those T_M ($CD62L^-CCR7^-$) circulating between blood and peripheral non-lymphoid tissues are known are "effector" T_M (T_{EM}). Nonetheless, besides their different location T_{CM} and T_{EM} cells also exhibit different phenotype and functional capacity suggesting that there is a division of labor between these two T_M populations. For instance, T_{CM} cells are self-renewing and produce high amounts of IL-2, maintaining the potential to differentiate into effector phenotypes after re-stimulation. In contrast, T_{EM} cells undergo limited homeostatic turnover, express tissue-homing factors and already exhibit an effector-like phenotype, such as the capacity to produce IFN-γ and TNF [52, 53]. Interestingly, there is a subgroup of T_{EM} that are derived from progenitors that enter the tissue during the effector phase which do not egress this compartment. These T_{EM} are also known as T_{RM} and they have lost the ability to recirculate via the blood [54-56].

TISSUE-RESIDENT MEMORY T CELLS (T_{RM})

$CD8^+$ T_{RM} cells are classically characterized by the expression of the early leukocyte activation marker CD69 and the integrin CD103 and play an important role in the control of local infections [57-60].

The down-regulation of the sphingosine-1-phosphate receptor (S1P1), which mediates cell egress from lymphoid tissues through the efferent lymphatics, is part of the transcriptional program that T_{EM} cells initiate in order to accumulate in peripheral tissues and become long-lived T_{RM} [53, 61, 62]. CD69 physically interacts with S1P1, an interaction that results in the inhibition and degradation of S1P1 preventing the departure of T cells from the infiltrating tissue [63, 64]. Indeed, $CD69^{-/-}$ $CD8^+$ T cells are unable to become T_{RM} since they fail to populate the skin and lung epitheliums [65, 66].

The expression of CD103 is thought to favor the retention of T cells in peripheral tissues by their interaction with its primary epithelial ligand E-cadherin, which is highly expressed by keratinocytes and Langerhans cells in the skin [67]. Hence, $CD103^+$ T_{RM} cells are mainly found in the epithelium of several tissues such as small intestine, salivary glands, heart, pancreas, kidney and skin [52, 53, 59]. The precise location of $CD103^+$ T_{RM} is intrinsically linked to the capacity of the tissue to secrete transforming growth factor-β (TGF-β), which is required for the expression of the integrin on the surface of $CD8^+$ T cells [65, 68-70].

Although CD69 and CD103 have been widely used to define T_{RM} cells in many compartments, recently several T_{RM} subsets have been identified that do not express these classic markers but fulfill the requirements to be considered long-lasting resident memory T cells. For example, $CD103^-$ T_{RM} are found in the secondary lymphoid tissues, small intestine, and liver [71-74], and double negatives ($CD69^-CD103^-$) represent approximately 60% of the T_{RM} in the female reproductive tract [75]. Accordingly, the expression of CD103 is tissue-dependent and the maintenance of $CD69^-$ T_{RM} could be mediated by alternative routes which in turn down-regulate S1P1, such as the zinc-finger transcription factor KLF-2 dependent-pathway [62].

Therefore, T_{RM} do not represent a homogenous population with a unique phenotypic signature, but a more complex community that shares the capacity to populate non-lymphoid tissues for long periods of time contributing to peripheral surveillance against secondary challenges.

CD8+ T CELLS IN THE SKIN

Healthy human skin contains approximately $1.1x10^6$ T cells per cm^3 which means that the body surface contains approximately twice the number of T cells than the entire circulatory system [76]. The majority of CD8+ T cells in the skin are localized in the epidermis in close contact with Langerhans cells. In humans, these CD8+ T cells predominantly express an αβ TCR, however in the mouse they predominantly express a γδ TCR [77, 78]. Interestingly, under resting conditions the majority of CD8+ T cells in the skin are T_{EM} and co-express CLA, CCR4 and CCR6 [4]. Human skin explant and parabiotic mice studies have demonstrated that 98% of CLA+ T_{EM} cells are in fact non-recirculating T_{RM} [4, 55]. Recently, it has been shown that the progenitor of these epithelial CD103+CD8+ T_{RM} cells lacks the expression of the effector marker killer cell lectin-like receptor subfamily G member 1 (KLRG1). The comparison of the transcriptional profiles of cutaneous T_{RM} and blood T_{CM} cells has shown that both populations share the same precursor which progressively acquires tissue-specific features to give rise to two T cell memory populations with distinct roles in protective immunity [53]. Part of this specialization program is the expression of the CD69 and CD103 surface markers in order to prevent emigration from the skin and to promote the retention of the T cells in this compartment, respectively [53, 67]. Skin long-lived memory T cells reside predominantly within the hair follicle epithelium which in turns favors the recruitment and formation of T_{RM} cells by the secretion of IL-15 and IL-17 [53, 79].

POSITIVE EFFECTS OF CD8+ T CELLS IN THE SKIN

Due to their strategic position in the epidermis, T_{RM} are relevant not only for the maintenance of skin immune homeostasis but also for the control of skin infections and malignancies.

Skin wound healing is a complex process that includes blood clotting, inflammatory cell recruitment, epithelial growth and tissue remodeling. In mice, γδ CD8+ T cells, also known as dendritic epidermal T cells (DETC), contribute to several stages of this process by secreting growth factors and chemokines [80]. After the recognition of antigen released by injured keratinocytes, murine DETCs produce insulin-like growth factor 1 (IGF-1) which is required by keratinocytes during development and maintenance [81].

Similar to murine γδ $CD8^+$ T cells, in humans both γδ and αβ activated skin $CD8^+$ T cells are able to secret IGF-1 in acute wounds. However, isolated T cells from skin chronic injures failed to produce pro-healing molecules upon further stimulation, suggesting that the over-exposure to persistent antigen might led to exhaustion and malfunction of these T cell subsets [82].

The protective role of cutaneous T_{RM} cells during secondary infections has been largely documented. The fact that in humans between 50 to 80% of herpes simplex virus (HSV) reinfections are resolved within 6 to 12 hours emphasizes the relevance of a preexistent local immune control [83]. After the resolution of HSV-2 infection, a population of long-lived antigen specific $CD8^+$ T cells remains in the interphase between the epidermis and dermis in close proximity to the peripheral nerves [84]. Interestingly, the phenotypic characterization of persistent $CD8^+$ T_{RM} at the site of previous HSV-2 infection showed that they belong to the CD8αα linage and upon activation they are able to produce cytolytic granules in order limit HSV-2 shedding and morbidity [85]. Work in mice has demonstrated that sterile inflammation in the skin is enough to trigger site-specific recruitment of activated $CD8^+$ T cells, the up-regulation of the integrin CD103 on their surface and ultimately their transformation into T_{RM} in the absence of antigen stimulation. Moreover, these epidermal T_{RM} subsets exerted superior protection against HSV-1 challenge compared to their circulating T_{CM} equivalents [86]. Recently, it has been proposed that although the initial activation of T_{RM} depends on the recognition of the cognate antigen via T cell receptor, the transcriptional profile down-stream once activated results in the secretion of a wide-range of antimicrobial molecules, including IFN-γ, which allow T_{RM} to be protective against a less specific but broader pathogen array [57].

It is well established and generally accepted that numerous members of the innate and adaptive immune responses participate in the recognition and destruction of cancer cells. After transformation, malignant cells express tumor-associated antigens on their surface that can activate cytotoxic tumor-specific T cells either by direct recognition via MHC class I or via specialized antigen-presenting cells (APCs), including dendritic cells (DCs) [87]. Th1 immune responses, characterized by the expression of IFN-γ and TNF, have been shown to be necessary to eradicate cancer cells. Conversely, Th2-driven responses that led to the secretion of immune suppressive cytokines, such as IL-4, IL-5, IL-10 and IL-13, are strongly correlated with tumor persistence and poor prognosis [88]. Experiments in transgenic γδ- or αβ $CD8^+$ T cell deficient mice have demonstrated that the absence of γδ T cells in the skin increased tumor development susceptibility upon exposure to chemical carcinogens or infusion of melanoma cell lines compared to their αβ-counterparts. In fact, the administration of a higher dose of carcinogen to αβ $CD8^+$ T cell deficient mice did not result in an increased detrimental effect, but in contrast, lead to a reduced susceptibility compared to wild-type animals, suggesting that skin αβ $CD8^+$ T cells might exert a negative effect on the generation of skin tumors [89, 90]. In subsequent studies, the efficacy of human γδ T cells in the control of skin tumor progression was assessed by using humanized mouse models in which human stem cells are adoptively transferred into severe combined immunodeficiency (SCID) mice in order to recreate the human immune system [91]. This mouse model demonstrated that human γδ $CD8^+$ T cells have significant antitumor activity against melanoma establishment and growth, however, the mechanism by which these cells favored the reduction of these tumors is still unknown [92].

Pathogenic Effects of $CD8^+$ T Cells in the Skin

Many cutaneous disorders arise as a direct consequence of dysregulation of the immune system in the skin. Psoriasis is a good example of a T cell mediated autoimmune disease. The main subset of T cells found in psoriatic lesions is CLA^+ and produces cytokines belonging to the Th1 repertoire. Therapies directed against Th1 products, such as monoclonal antibodies against TNF, or immunotherapies designed to skew Th1 response towards Th2, have been shown to be quite effective in the treatment of this disease [93-96]. The direct effect of tissue resident T cells on the development of this immunopathology was demonstrated by the fact that the xenotransplantation of healthy skin from psoriatic patients onto immune deficient mice resulted in the spontaneous development of psoriasis lesions. Moreover, local proliferation of resident human $CD8^+$ T cells was required for progression towards these malignant changes, since inhibiting T cell activation with monoclonal anti–human CD3 antibody muromonab-CD3 (OKT3) stopped the appearance of new lesions on the grafted skin [97]. Additionally, blocking the interaction between collagen and α1β1 integrin (VLA-1), which is specifically expressed on epidermal but not dermal T cells, prevented $CD8^+$ T cell skin retention and the subsequent psoriasis development [98].

Vitiligo is a skin disorder characterized by partial or total depigmentation of the epidermis. This disorder is triggered by the activation of skin antigen specific CD8+ T cells generated against melanocyte antigens, and results in the progressive and selective attack of melanocytes in the interfollicular epidermis and hair follicles [99]. Isolated auto-reactive T cells from vitiligo patients are able to recognize and trigger the apoptosis of healthy melanocytes *in vitro* [100, 101]. Interestingly, high numbers of cytotoxic CD8+ T cells with a Th1 cytokine profile are found in vitiligo lesions, where IFN-γ production seems to drive the activation of autoimmune cytotoxic T cells and the destruction of melanocytes [102, 103].

A Potential Role for CD8+ T Cells in the Regression of Precancerous SCC Lesions

From the clinical perspective, squamous cell carcinomas (SCC) comprise of cancers which originate from the squamous epithelium that covers organs such as skin, gastrointestinal tract, lungs and cervix [104]. The most frequent SCC are cutaneous, esophageal, non-small cell lung cancer and head and neck SCC, the latter of which includes the lips, oral and nasal cavities, paranasal sinuses, pharynx, larynx and parotid glands [104]. Non-melanoma skin cancers, which include cutaneous SCC and basal cell carcinoma (BCC), are the most common cancers in the Caucasian population with over 700,000 newly diagnosed cases each year in the United States. Although cutaneous SCC accounts for only 20% of the total non-melanoma skin cancer burden, it has a higher risk of metastasis compared to BCC, which makes prompt diagnosis and treatment crucial to avoid disease progression [105]. Ultra-violet (UV) radiation from the sun plays a key role in the establishment of SCC by causing DNA damage and mutations that in turn affect important anti-tumor checkpoints such as p53 [106, 107].

Precancerous SCC lesions in the skin, including Actinic Keratosis (AK), Bowen's Disease and Intraepithelial Carcinoma (IEC), undergo a high rate of spontaneous regression. Mutated p53 and the expression of cancer-testis antigens may provide CD8+ T cell target epitopes [108, 109], polyclonal CD8+ tumour infiltrating lymphocytes (TIL) are known to be present within AK and SCC lesions, and TILs derived from SCC lesions have been demonstrated to be cytotoxic for autologous tumour cell targets [110]. Nevertheless, precancerous lesions are frequently treated with immunomodulatory medications in order to prevent their potential progression to SCC. One such medication is imiquimod, a Toll-Like Receptor (TLR)-7/8 agonist. The mechanism through which imiquimod induces the regression of precancerous SCC lesions is not well understood, and as a consequence the immune outcomes of imiquimod application have been studied in various contexts over many years. In mice, the topical treatment of UV-induced SCC with imiquimod has been described to induce $CD8^+$ T cell, Th17 T cell, and pDC infiltration, and the up-regulation of mRNA for IL-12/23p40, Il-12p35, IL23p19, IL17A and IFN-γ [111]. In humans, the topical application of imiquimod is thought to target TLR-7 expression on Plasmacytoid Dendritic Cells (pDC) leading to the production of IFN-α and the expression of numerous IFN-α-inducible genes, including CIG5, IRF7, OAS1, OAS2, STAT1, MxA, MxB, IFI44, IFIT1, IFI35, IDG20, and GIP2 [112, 113]. More recently, a second mechanism of action has been attributed to the inflammation induced by the topical application of imiquimod. Imiquimod itself constitutes 5% of the pharmaceutical preparation of imiquimod known as Aldara. However, the second most abundant component in Aldara after water is in fact isostearic acid, which has been shown to promote keratinocyte inflammasome activation and induce keratinocyte death by pyroptosis (Caspase-1-dependent lysis), and lead to the release of IL-1α [114]. In addition to the induction of a strong inflammatory reaction Imiquimod treatment also results in substantial immune cell, including $CD8^+$ T cell, infiltration into multiple types of neoplasia in humans, including melanoma in situ, melanoma metastasis, precancerous SCC lesions, SCC, and Basal Cell Carcinoma (BCC) [112, 115, 116]. However, not all of these neoplasia's regress as a result of imiquimod treatment, so clearly $CD8^+$ T cell infiltration alone is not evidence of regression causality.

Mouse models are enormously useful when elucidating the mechanistic role of $CD8^+$ T cells in SCC regression. Over 40 years ago, *Kripke* demonstrated that SCC are highly immunogenic tumors which typically do not establish when transplanted into immune competent mice [117]. More recently, *Girardi and colleagues* confirmed this observation, but also demonstrated that a chemically-induced transplantable SCC cell line, PDV, will establish with high reproducibility in various T cell deficient mouse lines [118]. These include $TCR\beta^{-/-}$ (lacks all αβ T cells), $CD4^{-/-}$ (lacks $CD4^+$ T cells), and $\beta_2m^{-/-}$ (lacks $CD8^+$ T cells). Furthermore, the adoptive transfer of lymphocytes from immunoprotected wild-type mice (i.e., from mice previously challenged with PDV cells) into $TCR\beta^{-/-}$ mice conferred protection against SCC establishment. However, protection was not conferred if the lymphocytes were depleted of $CD4^+$ T cells or $CD8^+$ T cells prior to transfer. Mice deficient in IFN-γ also permitted the establishment of SCC, highlighting key roles for $CD8^+$ T cells, $CD4^+$ T cells, and IFN-γ in the prevention of (chemically-induced) SCC establishment in mice [118].

IMMUNOSUPPRESSION AND SCC DEVELOPMENT

The risk of developing SCC is greatly increased in patients rendered immunodeficient by disease or medication [119, 120]. Renal transplant recipients often receive triple therapy with combinations of Glucocorticoids (prednisolone or prednisone), calcineurin inhibitors (cyclosporine or tacrolimus) and anti-proliferative agents (azathioprine or mycophenolic acid) to prevent rejection of their allografts [121]. Worldwide, these patients suffer a 65-250 fold increased risk of non-melanoma skin cancer (NMSC) development compared with the general population [122, 123]. A single follow-up study of renal transplant recipients in Queensland, Australia, reported increased NMSC incidence with increasing duration of immunosuppression; over 50% developing at least one tumour within 10 years of immunosuppression [122]. Some renal transplant patients currently presenting to the Princess Alexandra Hospital, Brisbane, require the removal of ~120 primary skin tumours each year.

In order to try and gain insight into the connection between immune suppression and SCC incidence, numerous studies have compared the immune infiltrate of SCC in organ transplant patients (OTRs) with SCC arising in immune competent patients using established and emerging techniques [124]. *Walter and colleagues* utilised RT-PCR and immunohistochemical analysis to compare cancer-testis antigen expression, MHC class I expression, and $CD8^+$ T cell abundance in these two patient cohorts [108]. They reported that there was no difference in the proportion of patients expressing cancer-testis antigens or the number of different cancer-testis antigens expressed, and no differences in MHC class I staining, yet there was a reduction in $CD8^+$ T cell numbers in the intratumoral, peritumoral, and invasive regions in OTR SCC [108]. Their findings corroborated those of *Mühleisen and colleagues*, who, through the use of similar techniques reported a reduction in $CD8^+$ T cell proportions in the perineoplastic inflammatory infiltrate of OTR intraepithelial and invasive SCC [125]. However, in contrast to these findings, two studies from other groups have reported that the $CD8^+$ T cell density in OTR peritumoral infiltrates is not different to that in immune competent peritumoral infiltrates [126, 127]. Importantly, one of these studies, conducted by *Kosmidis and colleagues*, confirmed their immunohistochemical observations using RNA expression analysis. While levels of CD4, T-BET, IFN-γ, and IL-17A mRNA appeared reduced in OTRs, CD8 mRNA levels did not differ significantly between groups [126]. The literature therefore stands divided as to whether there are differences in $CD8^+$ T cell numbers in SCC following immunosuppression, but seems united as a whole that $CD8^+$ T cells are present. Thus, impaired recruitment of $CD8^+$ T cells does not appear to be the underlying factor contributing to SCC abundance in OTRs. This has led us, and others, to speculate that future studies should focus on a closer examination of $CD8^+$ T cell *function* as oppose to *abundance* in order to define the contribution of $CD8^+$ T cells to SCC abundance in OTRs [120, 127, 128].

$CD8^+$ T Cell Regulation in SCC

As highlighted previously, imiquimod is commonly used to induce the regression of precancerous SCC lesions. SCC, by contrast, displays a low clinical response rate to Imiquimod, and Imiquimod is therefore not recommended for the treatment of SCC [129]. This would seem surprising given studies that clearly show that imiquimod causes T cell infiltration into SCC. Indeed, *Smith* et al., treated SCC with Imiquimod for 7 days prior to excision and immunohistochemical analysis, and found that $CD8^+$ T cells, which represented 10-20% of the total T cell infiltrate in untreated SCC, represented 30-50% of all mononuclear cells post imiquimod treatment [130]. Furthermore, 60% of these $CD8^+$ T cells are were granzyme B-positive, suggesting they were primed for cytotoxic activity [130]. In a separate study, $CD8^+$ T cells from excised imiquimod-treated SCC were shown to produce more IFN-γ, granzyme, and perforin, and less IL-10 and TGF-β than $CD8^+$ T cells from untreated tumours [131]. In addition, imiquimod-treated SCC showed evidence of tumour cell apoptosis and histological evidence of tumor regression [131]. However, just why excised imiquimod-treated SCC show evidence of heightened $CD8^+$ T cell activity and tumour regression, yet non-excised imiquimod-treated SCC show a poor clinical response rate, is not well understood.

It has been proposed that SCC evade immune destruction by down-regulation of vascular E-selectin and recruitment of T-regs [132]. E-selectin down-regulation may be linked to the production of Nitric Oxide by Myeloid-Derived Suppressor Cells [133], however it should be noted that while imiquimod treatment increases vascular E-selectin expression [132], this does not appear to lead to SCC destruction *in vivo*. Another possibility is that antigen-presenting cells within SCC are somehow defective, and there is some evidence to suggest that dermal myeloid dendritic cells are deficient in their ability to stimulate T cells and that Langerhans cells are significantly decreased in number in SCC [134, 135]. However, a recent study showed that Langerhans cells isolated from human SCC are functional and may even be stronger at stimulating allogenic T cell responses than Langerhans cells from peritumoral skin [136]. Interestingly, tumour supernatant was found to enhance, rather than suppress, Langerhans cell-driven functional outcomes and Th1 bias despite the presence of immunosuppressive cytokines [136].

Recently, T-reg in SCC have been investigated to determine whether they play a role in permitting SCC growth and survival. We performed a flow-cytometry-based immunophenotypic screen of IEC and SCC lesions in immune competent patients and found that the relative abundance of $CD8^+$ T cells decreased with advancing disease stage [137]. Unexpectedly however, the relative abundance of $CD4^+FOXP3^+$ cells as a proportion of the total $CD3^+CD4^+$ T cell population did not change [137]. These results would appear to be corroborated by *Lai* et al., (2016; IHC, AK vs. SCC) and *Azzimonti* et al., (2015; IHC, well differentiated G1 SCC vs. more advanced moderately to poorly differentiated SCC G2-G3) [138, 139]. It should be noted, however, that in humans FOXP3 expression alone is not a good marker of T-regs as it can also be upregulated by activated T cells [140-142]. Subsequently, when *Azzimonti and colleagues* evaluated $FOXP3^+$ staining in concert with $CD25^+$ staining to identify $FOXP3^+CD25^+$ T-regs, they found that the abundance of T-regs was significantly increased in the peritumoral and intratumoral regions of G2-G3 SCC compared with G1 SCC [139]. T-reg analysis in humans is limited to correlative and/or observational studies, and so a functional role for $FOXP3^+CD25^+$ T-reg in the prevention of $CD8^+$ T cell-mediated SCC regression *in vivo* is difficult to define. Nevertheless, two recent and important studies have investigated the effects of T-regs on $CD8^+$ T cell *function* in the context of SCC. In a mouse model of chemically-induced SCC, *Serrels* et al., examined $FOXP3^+CD25^+$ T-reg abundance in wild-type SCC as compared with SCC lacking Focal Adhesion Kinase (FAK) [143]. FAK is a tyrosine kinase that regulates the transcription of inflammatory cytokines and chemokines leading to an immunosuppressive, pro-tumorigenic environment. SCC lacking FAK were shown to contain significantly fewer $FOXP3^+CD25^+$ T-reg and become susceptible to $CD8^+$ T cell-mediated regression. Furthermore, the treatment of palpable wild-type SCC with a FAK inhibitor, VS-4718, lead to a significant reduction in the abundance of $FOXP3^+CD25^+$ T-reg and CD8$^+$ T cell-mediated SCC regression [143]. Using co-cultures of highly purified patient SCC-derived CD25^{high}CD127^{low} T-reg and CD3$^+$CD8$^+$ T cells, *Lai* et al., (2016), demonstrated that T-reg suppress the proliferation of tumour-derived CD8$^+$ T cells, and the IFN-γ secretion by tumour-derived effector T cells, in response to the mitogen phytohemagglutinin (PHA) [138]. Thus, T-reg appear to play a clear role in the regulation of CD8$^+$ T cells within SCC.

CONCLUSION

The skin is the body's first barrier against external insults. Actively, CD8$^+$ T cells play a critical role in the defense against pathogens and malignancies in this compartment. Investigating this population more deeply has led to the discovery of five phenotypically and functionally distinct CD8$^+$ T cell subsets: naive, effector, effector memory, central memory and resident memory CD8$^+$ T cells. Of these five populations, T_{RM}, is believed to account for more than 90% of skin CD8$^+$ T cells during the steady state. T_{RM} in the skin are defined by their non- or limited ability to recirculate via blood and their capacity to survive in the tissue for years without apparent antigen stimulation. Nonetheless, T_{RM} have been demonstrated to be highly efficient in limiting secondary infections. Interestingly, after activation with cognate antigen T_{RM} are able to express a broad range of regulatory and cytotoxic molecules that protect against antigen non-related pathogens. Ultimately, the pathogen-alert role that T_{RM} provide in the skin is antigen independent, therefore, T_{RM} are a bridge between the adaptive and the innate immune responses. Despite their important implications in pathogen control and skin maintenance, our knowledge of their individual functional roles in skin homeostasis, including how they are themselves regulated to avoid unwanted pathogenic outcomes, is still in its infancy. For example, what role if any do T_{RM} play in the emergence and/or regression of skin cancer? What are the key elements of CD8$^+$ T cell function altered by aging that explain the increased prevalence of non-melanoma skin cancer in aged individuals? How can we effectively therapeutically manipulate CD8$^+$ T cell function in the skin and which CD8$^+$ T cell subsets should we be focusing our attention on? Clearly there is a pressing need for further research into these questions, alongside many important related questions, if we are to fully elucidate the role of this key adaptive immune cell in the skin.

ACKNOWLEDGMENTS

We acknowledge support for this work through a University of Queensland Early Career Fellowship (JC), and Institutional support and a Perpetual Trustees Fellowship (JW).

REFERENCES

[1] Naik, S., et al., Compartmentalized control of skin immunity by resident commensals. *Science,* 2012. 337(6098): p. 1115-9.

[2] Belkaid, Y. and S. Naik, Compartmentalized and systemic control of tissue immunity by commensals. *Nature immunology*, 2013. 14(7): p. 646-53.

[3] Kupper, T. and R. Fuhlbrigge, Immune surveillance in the skin: mechanisms and clinical consequences. *Nature reviews. Immunology*, 2004. 4: p. 211-222.

[4] Clark, R. A., et al., The Vast Majority of CLA+ T Cells Are Resident in Normal Skin. *The Journal of Immunology*, 2006. 176: p. 4431-4439.

[5] Evans, C. H., et al., EWS-FLI-1-targeted cytotoxic T-cell killing of multiple tumor types belonging to the Ewing sarcoma family of tumors. *Clin Cancer Res,* 2012. 18(19): p. 5341-51.

[6] Wells, J. W., et al., Semi-allogeneic dendritic cells can induce antigen-specific T-cell activation, which is not enhanced by concurrent alloreactivity. *Cancer immunology, immunotherapy*: CII, 2007. 56(12): p. 1861-73.

[7] Wells, J. W., et al., Regulation of allergic airway inflammation by class I-restricted allergen presentation and CD8 T-cell infiltration. *The Journal of allergy and clinical immunology*, 2007. 119(1): p. 226-34.

[8] Wells, J. W., et al., Suppression of allergic airway inflammation and IgE responses by a class I restricted allergen peptide vaccine. *Mucosal immunology,* 2009. 2(1): p. 54-62.

[9] Ferreira, E., et al., Inflammatory cytokines induce a unique mineralizing phenotype in mesenchymal stem cells derived from human bone marrow. *The Journal of biological chemistry*, 2013. 288(41): p. 29494-505.

[10] Coleman, M. A., et al., Tolerance induction with gene-modified stem cells and immune-preserving conditioning in primed mice: restricting antigen to differentiated antigen-presenting cells permits efficacy. *Blood,* 2012.

[11] Doan, T., et al., Steady-state dendritic cells continuously inactivate T cells that escape thymic negative selection. *Immunology and cell biology,* 2009. 87(8): p. 615-22.

[12] Steptoe, R. J., et al., Cognate CD4+ help elicited by resting dendritic cells does not impair the induction of peripheral tolerance in CD8+ T cells. *J Immunol*, 2007. 178(4): p. 2094-103.

[13] Steptoe, R. J., J. M. Ritchie, and L. C. Harrison, Transfer of hematopoietic stem cells encoding autoantigen prevents autoimmune diabetes. *The Journal of clinical investigation*, 2003. 111(9): p. 1357-63.

[14] Kenna, T. J., R. Thomas, and R. J. Steptoe, Steady-state dendritic cells expressing cognate antigen terminate memory CD8+ T-cell responses. *Blood*, 2008. 111(4): p. 2091-100.

[15] Honda, T., Y. Miyachi, and K. Kabashima, Regulatory T cells in cutaneous immune responses. *J Dermatol Sci*, 2011. 63(2): p. 75-82.

[16] Mattarollo, S. R., et al., NKT cells inhibit antigen-specific effector CD8 T cell induction to skin viral proteins. *Journal of immunology*, 2011. 187(4): p. 1601-8.

[17] Goubier, A., et al., Invariant NKT Cells Suppress CD8(+) T-Cell-Mediated Allergic Contact Dermatitis Independently of Regulatory CD4(+) T Cells. *The Journal of investigative dermatology*, 2012.

[18] Wu, T., et al., Smad3-deficient CD11b(+)Gr1(+) myeloid-derived suppressor cells prevent allograft rejection via the nitric oxide pathway. *J Immunol*, 2012. 189(10): p. 4989-5000.

[19] McNally, A., et al., CD4+CD25+ regulatory T cells control CD8+ T-cell effector differentiation by modulating IL-2 homeostasis. *Proc Natl Acad Sci USA*, 2011. 108(18): p. 7529-34.

[20] Dubois, B., et al., Innate CD4+CD25+ regulatory T cells are required for oral tolerance and inhibition of CD8+ T cells mediating skin inflammation. *Blood,* 2003. 102(9): p. 3295-301.

[21] Maurer, M., et al., Critical role of IL-10 in the induction of low zone tolerance to contact allergens. *The Journal of clinical investigation*, 2003. 112(3): p. 432-9.

[22] Eljaafari, A., et al., Isolation of human CD4/CD8 double-positive, graft-versus-host disease-protective, minor histocompatibility antigen-specific regulatory t cells and of a novel HLA-DR7-restricted HY-specific CD4 clone. *J Immunol*, 2013. 190(1): p. 184-94.

[23] Overgaard, N. H., et al., CD4+/CD8+ double-positive T cells: more than just a developmental stage? *J Leukoc Biol*, 2015. 97(1): p. 31-38.

[24] Riquelme, P., et al., IFN-gamma-induced iNOS Expression in Mouse Regulatory Macrophages Prolongs Allograft Survival in Fully Immunocompetent Recipients. *Mol Ther*, 2013. 21(2): p. 409-22.

[25] Muller, A. J., et al., Chronic inflammation that facilitates tumor progression creates local immune suppression by inducing indoleamine 2,3 dioxygenase. *Proc Natl Acad Sci USA, 2008*. 105(44): p. 17073-8.

[26] Wang, X. Z., et al., Virus-specific CD8 T cells in peripheral tissues are more resistant to apoptosis than those in lymphoid organs. *Immunity,* 2003. 18(5): p. 631-42.

[27] Coleman, M. A., et al., Antigen-encoding bone marrow terminates islet-directed memory CD8+ T-cell responses to alleviate islet transplant rejection. *Diabetes,* 2016.

[28] Adams, A. B., et al., Heterologous immunity provides a potent barrier to transplantation tolerance. *The Journal of clinical investigation*, 2003. 111(12): p. 1887-95.

[29] Jiang, X., et al., Skin infection generates non-migratory memory CD8+ T(RM) cells providing global skin immunity. *Nature*, 2012. 483(7388): p. 227-31.

[30] Gebhardt, T., et al., Memory T cells in nonlymphoid tissue that provide enhanced local immunity during infection with herpes simplex virus. *Nature immunology*, 2009. 10(5): p. 524-30.

[31] Wakim, L. M., et al., Enhanced survival of lung tissue-resident memory CD8(+) T cells during infection with influenza virus due to selective expression of IFITM3. *Nature immunology*, 2013. 14(3): p. 238-45.

[32] Liu, L., et al., Epidermal injury and infection during poxvirus immunization is crucial for the generation of highly protective T cell-mediated immunity. *Nature medicine*, 2010. 16(2): p. 224-7.

[33] Gebhardt, T., et al., Peripheral tissue surveillance and residency by memory T cells. *Trends in immunology*, 2013. 34(1): p. 27-32.

[34] Gebhardt, T. and L. K. Mackay, Local immunity by tissue-resident CD8(+) memory T cells. *Front Immunol*, 2012. 3: p. 340.

[35] Ahmed, R. and D. Gray, Immunological memory and protective immunity: understanding their relation. *Science,* 1996. 272: p. 54-60.

[36] Heath, W. R. and F. R. Carbone, Tolerance and Immunity. *Immunology,* 2001. 19: p. 47-64.
[37] Weninger, W., et al., T Cells. 2001. 194.
[38] Sallusto, F., et al., Two subsets of memory T lymphocytes with distinct homing potentials and effector functions. *Nature,* 1999. 401: p. 708-712.
[39] Masopust, D., et al., Linked references are available on JSTOR for this article: *Preferential Localization of Effector Memory Cells in Nonlymphoid Tissue*. 2001. 291: p. 2413-2417.
[40] Badovinac, V. P., J. S. Haring, and J. T. Harty, Initial T Cell Receptor Transgenic Cell Precursor Frequency Dictates Critical Aspects of the CD8+ T Cell Response to Infection. *Immunity,* 2007. 26: p. 827-841.
[41] Springer, T.A., Traffic signals of lymphocyte recirculation and leucocyte emigration: The multistep p aradigm. *Cell,* 1994. 76: p. 301-314.
[42] Zhou, S., et al., Critical role for perforin-, Fas/FasL-, and TNFR1-mediated cytotoxic pathways in down-regulation of antigen-specific T cells during persistent viral infection. *J Virol*, 2002. 76: p. 829-840.
[43] Lertmemongkolchai, G., et al., Bystander activation of CD8+ T cells contributes to the rapid production of IFN-gamma in response to bacterial pathogens. *Journal of immunology* (Baltimore, Md.: 1950), 2001. 166: p. 1097-1105.
[44] Cahill, R. N. P., et al., Two Distinct Pools of Recirculating T Lymphocytes: Migratory Characteristics of Nodal and Intestinal T Lymphocytes. *The Journal of Experimental Medicine*, 1977. 145: p. 420-428.
[45] McDermott, M. R. and J. Bienenstock, Evidence for a common mucosal immunologic system. *J. Immunol.*, 1979. 122: p. 1892-1898.
[46] Andreas Radbruch, A.H.F.A.D.V.E.B.M.L.R.B.U.H.H.R.R.H.A.S., P- and E-selectin mediate recuitment of T-helper-1 but not T-helper-2 cells into inflmaed tissues. *Nature,* 1997. 385: p. 810-813.
[47] Reiss, Y., et al., CC chemokine receptor (CCR)4 and the CCR10 ligand cutaneous T cell-attracting chemokine (CTACK) in lymphocyte trafficking to inflamed skin. *The Journal of experimental medicine,* 2001. 194: p. 1541-1547.
[48] Berlin, C., et al., α4β7 integrin mediates lymphocyte binding to the mucosal vascular addressin MAdCAM-1. *Cell,* 1993. 74: p. 185-195.
[49] Briskin, M., et al., Human mucosal addressin cell adhesion molecule-1 is preferentially expressed in intestinal tract and associated lymphoid tissue. *The American journal of pathology*, 1997. 151: p. 97-110.

[50] Svensson, M., et al., CCL25 mediates the localization to the small-intestinal mucosa Rapid Publication. *Journal of Clinical Investigation*, 2002. 110: p. 1113-1121.
[51] Badovinac, V. P. and J. T. Harty, Programming, demarcating, and manipulating CD8+ T-cell memory. *Immunological Reviews*, 2006. 211: p. 67-80.
[52] Casey, K. A., et al., Antigen-independent differentiation and maintenance of effector-like resident memory T cells in tissues. *Journal of immunology* (Baltimore, Md.: 1950), 2012. 188: p. 4866-75.
[53] Mackay, L. K., et al., The developmental pathway for CD103(+)CD8+ tissue-resident memory T cells of skin. *Nature immunology*, 2013. 14: p. 1294-301.
[54] Homann, D., L. Teyton, and M. B. Oldstone, Differential regulation of antiviral T-cell immunity results in stable CD8+ but declining CD4+ T-cell memory. *Nature medicine*, 2001. 7: p. 913-919.
[55] Jiang, X., et al., Skin infection generates non-migratory memory CD8+ T(RM) cells providing global skin immunity. *Nature*, 2012. 483: p. 227-31.
[56] Masopust, D., et al., Dynamic T cell migration program provides resident memory within intestinal epithelium. *The Journal of experimental medicine,* 2010. 207: p. 553-64.
[57] Ariotti, S., et al., T cell memory. Skin-resident memory $CD8^+$ T cells trigger a state of tissue-wide pathogen alert. *Science* (New York, N.Y.), 2014. 346: p. 101-5.
[58] Hofmann, M. and H. Pircher, E-cadherin promotes accumulation of a unique memory CD8 T-cell population in murine salivary glands. *Proceedings of the National Academy of Sciences*, 2011. 108: p. 16741-16746.
[59] Masopust, D., et al., Cutting edge: gut microenvironment promotes differentiation of a unique memory CD8 T cell population. *Journal of immunology* (Baltimore, Md.: 1950), 2006. 176: p. 2079-83.
[60] Schenkel, J. M. and D. Masopust, Tissue-resident memory T cells. *Immunity,* 2014. 41: p. 886-897.
[61] Brown, M. N., et al., Chemoattractant receptors and lymphocyte egress from extralymphoid tissue: changing requirements during the course of inflammation. *Journal of immunology* (Baltimore, Md.: 1950), 2010. 185: p. 4873-4882.

[62] Skon, C. N., et al., Transcriptional downregulation of S1pr1 is required for the establishment of resident memory CD8+ T cells. *Nature immunology,* 2013. 14: p. 1285-93.

[63] Bankovich, A. J., L. R. Shiow, and J. G. Cyster, CD69 suppresses sphingosine 1-phosophate receptor-1 (S1P1) function through interaction with membrane helix 4, in *Journal of Biological Chemistry*. 2010. p. 22328-22337.

[64] Shiow, L. R., et al., CD69 acts downstream of interferon-alpha/beta to inhibit S1P1 and lymphocyte egress from lymphoid organs. *Nature,* 2006. 440: p. 540-544.

[65] Lee, Y.-T., et al., Environmental and antigen receptor-derived signals support sustained surveillance of the lungs by pathogen-specific cytotoxic T lymphocytes. *Journal of virology*, 2011. 85: p. 4085-94.

[66] Mackay, L. K., et al., CD69 Interference with Sphingosine- 1-Phosphate Receptor Function Regulates Peripheral T Cell Retention. *Journal of immunology* (Baltimore, Md.: 1950), 2015: p. 1-5.

[67] Suffia, I., et al., A Role for CD103 in the Retention of CD4+CD25+ Treg and Control of Leishmania major Infection. *The Journal of Immunology,* 2005. 174: p. 5444-5455.

[68] Kane, C. J. M., et al., Transforming growth factor-β1 localization in normal and psoriatic epidermal keratinocytes in situ. *Journal of Cellular Physiology, 1990.* 144: p. 144-150.

[69] Koyama, S. Y. and D. K. Podolsky, Differential expression of transforming growth factors alpha and beta in rat intestinal epithelial cells. *J Clin Invest*, 1989. 83: p. 1768-1773.

[70] Wang, D., et al., Regulation of CD103 expression by CD8+ T cells responding to renal allografts. *Journal of immunology* (Baltimore, Md.: 1950), 2004. 172: p. 214-21.

[71] Anderson, K. G., et al., Cutting Edge: Intravascular Staining Redefines Lung CD8 T Cell Responses. *The Journal of Immunology*, 2012. 189: p. 2702-2706.

[72] Bergsbaken, T. and M. J. Bevan, Proinflammatory microenvironments within the intestine regulate the differentiation of tissue-resident CD8+ T cells responding to infection. *Nature immunology*, 2015. 16: p. 406-14.

[73] Schenkel, J. M., K. A. Fraser, and D. Masopust, Cutting edge: resident memory CD8 T cells occupy frontline niches in secondary lymphoid organs. *Journal of immunology* (Baltimore, Md.: 1950), 2014. 192: p. 2961-4.

[74] Tse, S.-W., et al., Unique transcriptional profile of liver-resident memory CD8+ T cells induced by immunization with malaria sporozoites. *Genes and immunity*, 2013. 14: p. 302-9.

[75] Steinert, E. M., et al., Quantifying memory CD8 T cells reveals regionalization of immunosurveillance. *Cell,* 2015. 161: p. 737-749.

[76] Clark, R. A., et al., The vast majority of CLA+ T cells are resident in normal skin. *J Immunol*, 2006. 176(7): p. 4431-9.

[77] Foster, B. Y. C. A., et al., HUMAN EPIDERMAL T CELLS PREDOMINATELY BELONG TO THE LINEAGE EXPRESSING a /b T CELL RECEPTOR. *Journal of Experimental Medicine*, 1990. 171.

[78] Havran, W. L., Y. H. Chien, and J. P. Allison, Recognition of self antigens by skin-derived T cells with invariant gamma delta antigen receptors. *Science,* 1991. 252: p. 1430-1432.

[79] Adachi, T., et al., Hair follicle–derived IL-7 and IL-15 mediate skin-resident memory T cell homeostasis and lymphoma. *Nature Medicine*, 2015. 21: p. 1272-1279.

[80] Jameson, J., et al., A Role for Skin gamma delta T Cells in Wound Repair. *Science*, 2002. 296: p. 747-749.

[81] Sharp, L. L., et al., Dendritic epidermal T cells regulate skin homeostasis through local production of insulin-like growth factor 1. *Nature immunology*, 2005. 6: p. 73-79.

[82] Toulon, A., et al., A role for human skin-resident T cells in wound healing. *The Journal of experimental medicine*, 2009. 206: p. 743-750.

[83] Mark, K. E., et al., Rapidly cleared episodes of herpes simplex virus reactivation in immunocompetent adults. *J Infect Dis,* 2008. 198: p. 1141-1149.

[84] Zhu, J., et al., Virus-specific CD8+ T cells accumulate near sensory nerve endings in genital skin during subclinical HSV-2 reactivation. *The Journal of experimental medicine*, 2007. 204: p. 595-603.

[85] Zhu, J., et al., Immune surveillance by CD8αα+ skin-resident T cells in human herpes virus infection. *Nature,* 2013. 497: p. 494-7.

[86] Mackay, L. K., et al., Long-lived epithelial immunity by tissue-resident memory T (TRM) cells in the absence of persisting local antigen presentation. *Proceedings of the National Academy of Sciences of the United States of America*, 2012. 109: p. 7037-42.

[87] Deguine, J., et al., Intravital imaging reveals distinct dynamics for natural killer and CD8+ T cells during tumor regression. *Immunity,* 2010. 33: p. 632-644.

[88] Constant, S. L. and K. Bottomly, Induction of Th1 and Th2 CD4+ T cell responses: the alternative approaches. *Annual review of immunology,* 1997. 15: p. 297-322.
[89] Gao, Y., et al., Gamma delta T cells provide an early source of interferon gamma in tumor immunity. *Journal of Experimental Medicine*, 2003. 198: p. 433-442.
[90] Girardi, M., et al., Regulation of cutaneous malignancy by gammadelta T cells. *Science* (New York, N.Y.), 2001. 294: p. 605-609.
[91] Bankert, R. B., N.K. Egilmez, and S. D. Hess, Human-SCID mouse chimeric models for the evaluation of anti-cancer therapies, in *Trends in Immunology*. 2001. p. 386-393.
[92] Lozupone, F., et al., Effect of human natural killer and gammadelta T cells on the growth of human autologous melanoma xenografts in SCID mice. *Cancer research*, 2004. 64: p. 378-385.
[93] Asadullah, K., et al., IL-10 is a key cytokine in psoriasis: Proof of principle by IL-10 therapy: A new therapeutic approach. *Journal of Clinical Investigation*, 1998. 101: p. 783-794.
[94] Ghoreschi, K., et al., Interleukin-4 therapy of psoriasis induces Th2 responses and improves human autoimmune disease. *Nature medicine,* 2003. 9: p. 40-46.
[95] Trepicchio, W. L., et al., Interleukin-11 therapy selectively downregulates type I cytokine proinflammatory pathways in psoriasis lesions. *Journal of Clinical Investigation*, 1999. 104: p. 1527-1537.
[96] Williams, J. D. L. and C. E. M. Griffiths, Cytokine blocking agents in dermatology. *Clinical and Experimental Dermatology*, 2002. 27: p. 585-590.
[97] Boyman, O., et al., Spontaneous development of psoriasis in a new animal model shows an essential role for resident T cells and tumor necrosis factor-alpha. *J Exp Med*, 2004. 199: p. 731-736.
[98] Conrad, C., et al., Alpha1beta1 integrin is crucial for accumulation of epidermal T cells and the development of psoriasis. *Nature medicine*, 2007. 13: p. 836-842.
[99] Lotti, T. and A. M. D'Erme, Vitiligo as a systemic disease, in Clinics in Dermatology. 2014, Elsevier Inc. p. 430-434.
[100] Ogg, G. S., et al., High frequency of skin-homing melanocyte-specific cytotoxic T lymphocytes in autoimmune vitiligo. *The Journal of experimental medicine,* 1998. 188: p. 1203-8.

[101] Wańkowicz-Kalińska, A., et al., Immunopolarization of CD4+ and CD8+ T cells to Type-1-like is associated with melanocyte loss in human vitiligo. *Laboratory investigation; a journal of technical methods and pathology*, 2003. 83: p. 683-95.
[102] Harris, J. E., et al., A mouse model of vitiligo with focused epidermal depigmentation requires IFN-γ for autoreactive $CD8^+$ T-cell accumulation in the skin. *The Journal of investigative dermatology,* 2012. 132: p. 1869-76.
[103] van den Boorn, J. G., et al., Autoimmune destruction of skin melanocytes by perilesional T cells from vitiligo patients. *The Journal of investigative dermatology,* 2009. 129: p. 2220-2232.
[104] Markey, A. C., Etiology and pathogenesis of squamous cell carcinoma. *Clinics in Dermatology*, 1995. 13: p. 537-543.
[105] Clayman, G. L., et al., Mortality risk from squamous cell skin cancer. *J Clin Oncol*, 2005. 23(4): p. 759-65.
[106] Rodust, P. M., et al., UV-induced squamous cell carcinoma--a role for antiapoptotic signalling pathways. *The British journal of dermatology*, 2009. 161 Suppl p. 107-15.
[107] Shreedhar, V. K., et al., Origin and characteristics of ultraviolet-B radiation-induced suppressor T lymphocytes. *Journal of immunology* (Baltimore, Md.: 1950), 1998. 161: p. 1327-1335.
[108] Walter, A., et al., Cancer-testis antigens and immunosurveillance in human cutaneous squamous cell and basal cell carcinomas. *Clin Cancer Res,* 2010. 16(14): p. 3562-70.
[109] Black, A. P., et al., p53-specific CD8+ T-cell responses in individuals with cutaneous squamous cell carcinoma. *Br J Dermatol*, 2005. 153(5): p. 987-91.
[110] Haeffner, A. C., et al., Analysis of tumor-infiltrating lymphocytes in cutaneous squamous cell carcinoma. *Arch Dermatol*, 1997. 133(5): p. 585-90.
[111] Yokogawa, M., et al., Imiquimod attenuates the growth of UVB-induced SCC in mice through Th1/Th17 cells. *Mol Carcinog*, 2013. 52(10): p. 760-9.
[112] Urosevic, M., et al., Disease-independent skin recruitment and activation of plasmacytoid predendritic cells following imiquimod treatment. *J Natl Cancer Inst,* 2005. 97(15): p. 1143-53.
[113] Urosevic, M., et al., Imiquimod treatment induces expression of opioid growth factor receptor: a novel tumor antigen induced by interferon-alpha? *Clin Cancer Res*, 2004. 10(15): p. 4959-70.

[114] Walter, A., et al., Aldara activates TLR7-independent immune defence. *Nat Commun*, 2013. 4: p. 1560.

[115] Ooi, T., et al., Imiquimod-induced regression of actinic keratosis is associated with infiltration by T lymphocytes and dendritic cells: a randomized controlled trial. *Br J Dermatol*, 2006. 154(1): p. 72-8.

[116] Wolf, I. H., et al., Nature of inflammatory infiltrate in superficial cutaneous malignancies during topical imiquimod treatment. *Am J Dermatopathol,* 2007. 29(3): p. 237-41.

[117] Kripke, M. L., Antigenicity of murine skin tumors induced by ultraviolet light. *J Natl Cancer Inst*, 1974. 53(5): p. 1333-6.

[118] Girardi, M., et al., Characterizing the protective component of the alphabeta T cell response to transplantable squamous cell carcinoma. *J Invest Dermatol,* 2004. 122(3): p. 699-706.

[119] Wells, J. W., Do actinic keratoses and superficial squamous cell carcinomas have a specific immunoprofile? *Curr Probl Dermatol*, 2015. 46: p. 36-41.

[120] Jung, J. W., et al., Does the nature of residual immune function explain the differential risk of non-melanoma skin cancer development in immunosuppressed organ transplant recipients? *Int J Cancer*, 2016. 138(2): p. 281-92.

[121] Burke, M. T., et al., Genetics and nonmelanoma skin cancer in kidney transplant recipients. *Pharmacogenomics,* 2015. 16(2): p. 161-72.

[122] Ramsay, H. M., et al., Non-melanoma skin cancer risk in the Queensland renal transplant population. *Br J Dermatol*, 2002. 147(5): p. 950-6.

[123] Lindelof, B., et al., Incidence of skin cancer in 5356 patients following organ transplantation. *Br J Dermatol*, 2000. 143(3): p. 513-9.

[124] Cruz, J. L. and J. W. Wells, Assessing T-cell abundance in cutaneous squamous cell carcinoma: adding another string to your bow. *Exp Dermatol,* 2016.

[125] Muhleisen, B., et al., Progression of cutaneous squamous cell carcinoma in immunosuppressed patients is associated with reduced CD123+ and FOXP3+ cells in the perineoplastic inflammatory infiltrate. *Histopathology, 2009.* 55(1): p. 67-76.

[126] Kosmidis, M., et al., Immunosuppression affects CD4+ mRNA expression and induces Th2 dominance in the microenvironment of cutaneous squamous cell carcinoma in organ transplant recipients. J Immunother, 2010. 33(5): p. 538-46.

[127] Krynitz, B., B. Lundh Rozell, and B. Lindelof, Differences in the peritumoural inflammatory skin infiltrate between squamous cell carcinomas in organ transplant recipients and immunocompetent patients. Acta Derm Venereol, 2010. 90(4): p. 379-85.
[128] Rovira, J., et al., A color-coded reporter model to study the effect of immunosuppressants on CD8+ T-cell memory in antitumor and alloimmune responses. Transplantation, 2013. 95(1): p. 54-62.
[129] Love, W. E., J. D. Bernhard, and J. S. Bordeaux, Topical imiquimod or fluorouracil therapy for basal and squamous cell carcinoma: a systematic review. Arch Dermatol, 2009. 145(12): p. 1431-8.
[130] Smith, K. J., S. Hamza, and H. Skelton, Topical imidazoquinoline therapy of cutaneous squamous cell carcinoma polarizes lymphoid and monocyte/macrophage populations to a Th1 and M1 cytokine pattern. *Clin Exp Dermatol*, 2004. 29(5): p. 505-12.
[131] Huang, S. J., et al., Imiquimod enhances IFN-gamma production and effector function of T cells infiltrating human squamous cell carcinomas of the skin. *J Invest Dermatol*, 2009. 129(11): p. 2676-85.
[132] Clark, R. A., et al., Human squamous cell carcinomas evade the immune response by down-regulation of vascular E-selectin and recruitment of regulatory T cells. *J Exp Med*, 2008. 205(10): p. 2221-34.
[133] Gehad, A. E., et al., Nitric oxide-producing myeloid-derived suppressor cells inhibit vascular E-selectin expression in human squamous cell carcinomas. *J Invest Dermatol*, 2012. 132(11): p. 2642-51.
[134] Bluth, M. J., et al., Myeloid dendritic cells from human cutaneous squamous cell carcinoma are poor stimulators of T-cell proliferation. *J Invest Dermatol,* 2009. 129(10): p. 2451-62.
[135] Takahara, M., et al., Stromal CD10 expression, as well as increased dermal macrophages and decreased Langerhans cells, are associated with malignant transformation of keratinocytes. *J Cutan Pathol*, 2009. 36(6): p. 668-74.
[136] Fujita, H., et al., Langerhans cells from human cutaneous squamous cell carcinoma induce strong type 1 immunity. *J Invest Dermatol*, 2012. 132(6): p. 1645-55.
[137] Freeman, A., et al., Comparative immune phenotypic analysis of cutaneous Squamous Cell Carcinoma and Intraepidermal Carcinoma in immune-competent individuals: proportional representation of CD8+ T-cells but not FoxP3+ Regulatory T-cells is associated with disease stage. *PLoS One*, 2014. 9(10): p. e110928.

[138] Lai, C., et al., OX40+ Regulatory T Cells in Cutaneous Squamous Cell Carcinoma Suppress Effector T-Cell Responses and Associate with Metastatic Potential. *Clin Cancer Res*, 2016.

[139] Azzimonti, B., et al., Intense Foxp3+ CD25+ regulatory T-cell infiltration is associated with high-grade cutaneous squamous cell carcinoma and counterbalanced by CD8+/Foxp3+ CD25+ ratio. *Br J Dermatol*, 2015. 172(1): p. 64-73.

[140] Gavin, M. A., et al., Single-cell analysis of normal and FOXP3-mutant human T cells: FOXP3 expression without regulatory T cell development. *Proc Natl Acad Sci USA,* 2006. 103(17): p. 6659-64.

[141] Pillai, V., et al., Transient regulatory T-cells: a state attained by all activated human T-cells. *Clin Immunol*, 2007. 123(1): p. 18-29.

[142] Allan, S. E., et al., Activation-induced FOXP3 in human T effector cells does not suppress proliferation or cytokine production. *Int Immunol*, 2007. 19(4): p. 345-54.

[143] Serrels, A., et al., Nuclear FAK controls chemokine transcription, Tregs, and evasion of anti-tumor immunity. *Cell,* 2015. 163(1): p. 160-73.

In: Horizons in Cancer Research. Volume 63 ISBN: 978-1-53610-013-6
Editor: Hiroto S. Watanabe

Chapter 6

TRITERPENOIDS AS ANTI-CANCER AND REVERSAL AGENTS OF ABC TRANSPORTER-MEDIATED MDR IN CANCER

Pranav Gupta, Dong-Hua Yang and Zhe-Sheng Chen*
Department of Pharmaceutical Sciences, College of Pharmacy
and Health Sciences, St. John's University, Queens, New York, NY, US

ABSTRACT

Triterpenoids, often referred as terpenes, are compounds of natural and semi-synthetic origin containing a dual five carbon backbone. Triterpenoids have been documented as analgesic, anti-inflammatory, anti-viral, anti-microbial, hepatoprotective, sedative, and cardioprotective in a number of studies. In addition, triterpenoids have been extensively studied as potent anti-cancer agents. Anti-cancer mechanisms of triterpenoid action include blockade of nuclear factor (NF)-κB activation, induction of apoptosis, and suppression of angiogenesis causing mitochondrial dysfunction. Moreover, triterpenoids have been studied, pre clinically, as reversal agents of ABC transporter-mediated multi drug resistance (MDR) in cancer. They have been shown to block the efflux function of a multitude of drug efflux transporters, thereby causing an increase in drug accumulation and cell death. This chapter discusses our

*Corresponding author, Zhe-Sheng Chen, Department of Pharmaceutical Sciences, College of Pharmacy and Health Sciences, St. John's University, Queens, New York 11439, USA, Email: chenz@stjohns.edu, Phone: 1-718-990-1432, Fax: 1-718-990-1877.

current knowledge of the molecular basis of anti-cancer drug resistance and the mechanisms through which triterpenoids modulate ABC transporter-mediated MDR.

1. INTRODUCTION

Triterpenes are synthetic hydrocarbons composed of six isoprene units and as much as 30 carbon atoms [1]. Naturally occurring triterpenes are called triterpenoids. Till date, over 20,000 triterpenoids have been isolated and characterized from natural sources [1]. Triterpenoids are ubiquitous in nature, easily found in fungi, ferns, and marine sponges and form major constituent of many Chinese herbal medicines, such ginseng and *platycodon* [2]. Studies done so far have shown that triterpenoids have therapeutic effects against cancer, inflammation, liver toxicity, and cardiovascular diseases [2-4]. Figure 1 shows the mechanisms of triterpenoid action.

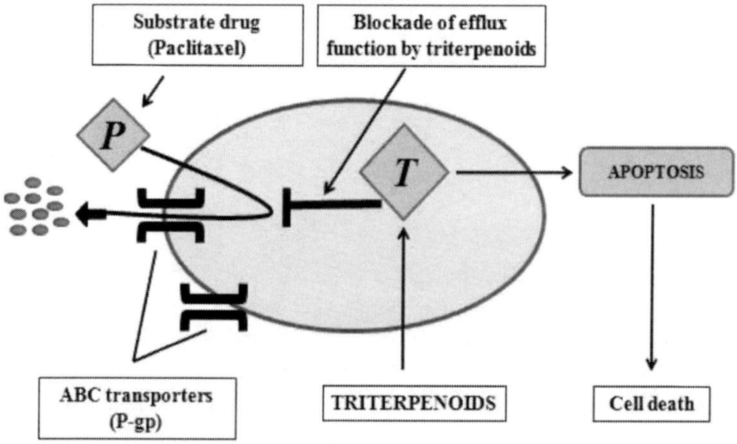

Figure 1. Mechanisms of triterpenoid action as anti-cancer and reversal agents of ABC transporter-mediated MDR in cancer. Chronic use of chemotherapeutic drugs causes cancer cells to develop drug resistance. Overexpression of ABC transporters, such as P-gp is one of the major causes of MDR. These transporters pump out substrate drugs, such as paclitaxel from cancer cells. In the presence of triterpenoids, the efflux function of ABC transporters is blocked, thereby increasing the intracellular accumulation of substrate drugs inside the cancer cells. Moreover, triterpenoids exerts cellular effects, such as induction of apoptosis and promotes cancer cell death.

2. Triterpenoids as Anti-Cancer Agents

Over the years, a number of studies have been conducted demonstrating the anti-cancer potentials of triterpenoids. Triterpenoids are cytotoxic to cancer cells and exhibit potent chemopreventive effects. The anti-tumorigenic effect of these agents is attributed to a number of mechanisms, such as blockade of inflammatory mediator (nuclear factor-κB), induction of apoptosis, inhibition of cell proliferation, suppression of angiogenesis, and mitochondrial dysfunction [5]. Primarily, three receptor types contribute towards the anti-cancer activity of triterpenoids, viz., androgen receptors, aryl hydrogen receptors, and the vascular endothelial growth factor (VEGF) family of receptors [1]. Some of the most potent triterpenoids as anti-cancer agents are discussed here and summarized in Table 1.

2.1. Avicins

Avicins are saponin triterpenoids isolated from the plant *Acaia victoriae* (family; leguminosae) [6]. Avicins are synthesized as a result of plant stress and have been known to suppress innate immunity responses [6]. Commercial production of avicins requires an extensive stress inducing model in *in vitro* plant cultures. Avicins inhibit nuclear localization and DNA binding of NF-κB, thus causing its inactivation [3, 7].

2.2. Betulin

Betulin, a pentacyclic triterpenoid, is isolated from the plant *Betula alba* [8].Pharmacologically, betulinic acid (a derivative of betulin) has found to be therapeutically active against different cancers, such as skin cancer and melanoma [8]. Moreover, anti-inflammatory and anti-viral effects of betulinic acid have been extensively studied [8, 9]. Studies have shown that betulinic acid suppresses IκBα kinase and p65 phosphorylation *in vitro*, thus inhibiting the carcinogen induced activation of NF-κB [9]. However, due to its inhibition of IKKα, betulinic acid may exert severe toxicity in pregnant women.

2.3. Ursolic Acid

Ursolic acid is a pentacyclic triterpene found in many herbal remedies. It has been used as an anti-inflammatory, anti-hyperlipidemic and anti-cancer agent [10]. Ursolic acid has been reported to inhibit the activation and phosphorylation of IκBα [11]. Moreover, it blocks p65 phosphorylation and DNA binding of NF-κB [11]. Therefore, ursolic acid has a dual action in preventing inflammation and inducing apoptosis in cancer cells.

2.4. CDDO-Me/I M

2-Cyano-3, 12-dioxoolean-1,9-dien-28- oic acid (CDDO), its C-28 methyl ester (CDDO-Me), and its C-28 imidazole (CDDO-Im) are synthetic forms of ursolic triterpenoids. These are reported to be potent anti-cancer agents. CDDO and its derivatives are known to inhibit solid tumors and leukemias. Unlike many other anti-cancer agents, CDDO and its derivatives do not affect the phosphorylation of p53. They cause cytotoxicity through the upregulation of cell cycle regulating proteins, viz; p21, p27, and cyclin D1. Furthermore, induction of reactive oxygen species by CDDO-Me has been reported to cause significant cytotoxicity in ovarian cancer cells. Moreover, CDDO-Me blocks Akt without altering the expression of PDK1 or 2.

Table 1. Triterpenoids as anti-cancer agents

S.No.	Compound	Mechanism of anti-cancer action	Therapeutic use
1)	Avicins	NF-κB inactivation	Cancer and inflammation
2)	Betulin	IKKα inhibition and NF-κB inactivation	Leukemia, Melanoma, and inflammation
3)	Ursolic acid	IKKα inhibition, NF-κB inactivation, and inhibition of p65 phosphorylation	Carcinogenesis and inflammation
4)	CDDO-Me/I m	Upregulation of cyclin dependent kinases, ROS production, and inhibition of Akt	Leukemia, Melanoma, and inflammation

3. Triterpenoids as Chemosensitizers against Multi-Drug Resistance (MDR) Efflux Pumps

Besides being potent anti-cancer agents, triterpenoids exhibit chemosensitizing properties against major drug efflux pumps. Triterpenoids, when combined with chemotherapeutic substrate drugs such as, paclitaxel, doxorubicin, mitoxantrone, vincristine and vinblastine, shows significant increase in cytotoxicity in both drug-sensitive and drug-resistant cancer cells [12].

Derivatives of betulinic, oleanolic and pomolic acids have been studied to overcome MDR in K562 human chronic myeloid leukemia cells [13]. Janaina et al. carried out the fractionalization of *Licania tomentosa* and *Chrysobalanus icaco* to isolate betulinic, oleanolic and pomolic acids [13]. These triterpenoids exhibited significant cytotoxicity against K562 cells and induced apoptosis [13]. Furthermore, their effect on modulating the MDR was evaluated using vincristine-resistant K562 cells [13]. These cells overexpressed ABCB1 (also known as P-glycoprotein) transporter which is one of the major causes of MDR in cancer cells. Interestingly, all three triterpenoids potently inhibited the growth of vincristine-resistant K562 cells, suggesting a possible blockade of the efflux function of ABCB1 multi-drug transporter [13]. Similarly, cycloartanes reversed MDR in L5178Y mouse lymphoma cells [14]. A significant increase in the intracellular accumulation of rhodamine 123 was observed when the resistant L5178Y cells were treated with the isolated cycloartanes [14]. A number of studies have reported the triterpenoid induced inhibition of drug efflux transporters viz. P-gp, BCRP, and MRP1.

3.1. Triterpenoids as Inhibitors of P-gp

P-gp, also known as ABCB1, is the first member of the subfamily B of ATP-binding cassette (ABC) transporters [15]. It is known to be the first ABC transporter discovered in humans [16]. P-gp is a 170-kDa transmembrane protein that is located in liver, kidneys, intestines, and blood- brain barrier [16, 17]. An ATP-dependent mechanism promotes efflux of drugs through P-gp, thus rendering less intracellular concentrations of the substrate drug [15-17].

Modulation of P-gp function has always been a major goal to combat MDR. Until now three generation of P-gp inhibitors have been identified to block the efflux function of this transporter. Verapamil, a calcium channel blocker, was the first P-gp inhibitor identified; however the high dose of verapamil limited its clinical applicability [18]. Drugs like valspodar, biricodar, and dexverapamil were categorized as the second generation of P-gp inhibitors [18, 19]. In clinics, these drugs showed pronounced pharmacokinetic interactions with other chemotherapeutic drugs, this lead to the search for safer drugs [19]. The third generation of P-gp modulators had relatively less pharmacokinetic interactions but clinically their toxicity is still a major concern [20].Over the years, researchers have explored the P-gp inhibitory function of a number of triterpenoids. Zhang et al. evaluated the P-gp reversal activity of two sipholenol analogs isolated from *Callyspongiasiphonella* [21]. At 5μM, both the analogs significantly reversed P-gp mediated MDR in drug resistant and transfected ABCB1 overexpressing cells. Moreover, these analogs did not affect the protein expression of ABCB1 and stimulated the intracellular accumulation of paclitaxel (a known substrate of ABCB1) [21]. Two other studies reported several other sipholenol analogs as potent inhibitors of P-gp mediated MDR [22, 23].

In 2014, Liu et al. reported the P-gp reversal activity of a cyclolanstane triterpenoid [24]. Acerinol is widely found in Chinese herbs such as *Cimicifuga acerina, Cimicifuga simplex, Cimicifuga japonica, and Cimicifuga yunnanensis* [25]. Acerinol was tested for its ability to inhibit the efflux function of P-gp in drug-sensitive and drug-resistant human hepatocellular carcinoma cell lines (HepG2 and HepG2/ADM) and human breast cancer cell lines (MCF-7 and MCF-7/ADR). Acerinol at 4 μM, increased the sensitivity of HepG2/ADM and MCF-7/ADR cells to doxorubicin, vincristine, and paclitaxel. Furthermore, acerinol increased the intracellular accumulation of doxorubicin and rhodamine 123 in drug-resistant cells without altering the protein expression of the transporter. Moreover, a stimulation of ATPase was observed suggesting that acerinol inhibits P-gp function in a competitive manner [24]. Another triterpenoid, ginsenoside Rg3 (a ginseng saponin) showed potent inhibition of P-gp function [26]. Rg3 increased the intracellular accumulation of rhodamine 123 and inhibited the efflux of radiolabeled substrate drug vinblastine from the drug-resistant KBV20C cells [26]. Similarly, derivatives of hydroxybetulinic acid [27] and extracts of *Poria cocos* [28] inhibited the efflux of substrate drugs from vincristine-resistant KBV200 cells. Table 2 summarizes triterpenoids as P-gp inhibitors.

3.2. Triterpenoids as Inhibitors of BCRP

BCRP, also known as ABCG2, is the second member of subfamily G of the ABC transporters [16]. BCRP is the first identified half transporter with a molecular weight of 72-kDa [15]. It is present in placenta, liver, intestines, and veins and capillaries of blood vessels [15-17]. Common substrates of ABCG2 include tyrosine kinase inhibitors (TKIs), anthracyclines, methotrexate, and camptothecin-derived topoisomerase I inhibitors [15, 16]. Yoshida et al. screened seven triterpenoids for their reversal activity against BCRP [29]. They carried out the transport studies using membrane vesicles obtained from BCRP overexpressing LLC-PK1 cells [29]. Amongst the seven triterpenoids tested, glycyrrhetic acid showed maximum transport of substrate drug ($E_2 17\beta G$) through BCRP membrane vesicles as compared to the control [29]. However, the exact mechanism of triterpenoid-mediated BCRP inhibition and its effect on the ATPase activity of BCRP still needs to be elucidated.

3.3. Triterpenoids as Inhibitors of MRP1

MRP1, also known as ABCC1, is the first member of subfamily C of the ABC transporters [30]. It is a 190-kDa protein present mostly on the basolateral surface of the epithelial membrane [16, 30]. Overexpression of MRP1 confers resistance to methotrexate, camptothecins, anthracyclines, vinca alkaloids, and mitoxantrone [15, 16]. Braga et al. reported the inhibition of MRP1 by oleanolic acid in Ma104 monkey kidney embryo cells [31]. Oleanolic acid at 10 μg/ml increased the intracellular accumulation of CFDA (carboxy-fluorescein diacetate) [31]. CFDA is a substrate drug used for colorimetric measurement of ABCC1 activity. Moreover, there was no change in the protein expression and mRNA levels of MRP1 when Ma104 cells were treated with oleanolic acid suggesting that it affects the function and not the structure of MRP1 [31].

Unlike P-gp, triterpenoid-mediated MRP1 inhibition has been less studied and a few hypotheses exist for their possible inhibitory mechanism: 1) triterpenoid may decrease the intracellular concentrations of glutathione (GSH) required for MRP1 function [32], 2) allosteric interaction of triterpenoids and MRP1 [4], and 3) a slight modulation of MRP1 expression [2, 4].

Table 2. Triterpenoids as reversal agents of multi-drug resistant efflux pumps

S.No.	Compound	Increased accumulation of substrate drug	Major ABC transporter inhibited
1)	Sipholenol analogs	Paclitaxel	P-gp
2)	Acerinol	Doxorubicin and rhodamine 123	P-gp
3)	Ginsenoside	Rhodamine 123 and vinblastine	P-gp
4)	Hydroxybetulinic acid derivatives	Vincristine	P-gp and BCRP
5)	Glycyrrhetic acid	$E_2 17\beta G$	BCRP
6)	Oleanolic acid	CFDA, rhodamine 123	MRP1

CONCLUSION

Extensive research done in the past provides evidence of the development of triterpenoids for cancer prevention and treatment. Both natural and semi-synthetic triterpenoids have been explored for their vast majority of therapeutic effects. Triterpenoids have successfully been evaluated in both *in vitro* and *in vivo* models as anti-cancer and reversal agents; however their clinical significance is still questionable. Having discussed their therapeutic potentials in this chapter, further development of triterpenoids demands the concern of bioavailability, pharmacodynamics, toxicity and tumor eradication to be addressed.

Conflict of Interest

The authors declare no conflict of interest.

REFERENCES

[1] Salminen A, Lehtonen M, Suuronen T, Kaarniranta K, Huuskonen J. Terpenoids: natural inhibitors of NF-kappaB signaling with anti-inflammatory and anticancer potential. *Cell Mol Life Sci.* 2008;65(19):2979-99.

[2] Yan XJ, Gong LH, Zheng FY, Cheng KJ, Chen ZS, Shi Z. Triterpenoids as reversal agents for anticancer drug resistance treatment. *Drug DiscovToday*. 2014;19(4):482-8.

[3] Haridas V, Arntzen CJ, Gutterman JU. Avicins, a family of triterpenoid saponins from Acacia victoriae (Bentham), inhibit activation of nuclear factor-kappaB by inhibiting both its nuclear localization and ability to bind DNA. *Proc Natl Acad Sci USA*. 2001;98(20):11557-62.

[4] Wu CP, Calcagno AM, Hladky SB, Ambudkar SV, Barrand MA. Modulatory effects of plant phenols on human multidrug-resistance proteins 1, 4 and 5 (ABCC1, 4 and 5). *FEBS J*. 2005;272(18):4725-40.

[5] Molnár J, Gyémánt N, Tanaka M, Hohmann J, Bergmann-Leitner E, Molnár P, et al. Inhibition of multidrug resistance of cancer cells by natural diterpenes, triterpenes and carotenoids. *Curr Pharm Des*. 2006;12(3):287-311.

[6] Haridas V, Hanausek M, Nishimura G, Soehnge H, Gaikwad A, Narog M, et al. Triterpenoid electrophiles (avicins) activate the innate stress response by redox regulation of a gene battery. *J Clin Invest*. 2004;113(1):65-73.

[7] Haridas V, Kim SO, Nishimura G, Hausladen A, Stamler JS, Gutterman JU. Avicinylation (thioesterification): a protein modification that can regulate the response to oxidative and nitrosative stress. *Proc Natl AcadSci USA*. 2005;102(29):10088-93.

[8] Alakurtti S, Mäkelä T, Koskimies S, Yli-Kauhaluoma J. Pharmacological properties of the ubiquitous natural product betulin. *Eur J Pharm Sci*. 2006;29(1):1-13.

[9] Takada Y, Aggarwal BB. Betulinic acid suppresses carcinogen-induced NF-kappa B activation through inhibition of I kappa B alpha kinase and p65 phosphorylation: abrogation of cyclooxygenase-2 and matrix metalloprotease-9. *J Immunol*. 2003;171(6):3278-86.

[10] Liu J. Pharmacology of oleanolic acid and ursolic acid. *J Ethnopharmacol*. 1995;49(2):57-68.

[11] Shishodia S, Majumdar S, Banerjee S, Aggarwal BB. Ursolic acid inhibits nuclear factor-kappaB activation induced by carcinogenic agents through suppression of IkappaBalpha kinase and p65 phosphorylation: correlation with down-regulation of cyclooxygenase 2, matrix metalloproteinase 9, and cyclin D1. *Cancer Res.* 2003;63(15):4375-83.
[12] Abraham I, El Sayed K, Chen ZS, Guo H. Current status on marine products with reversal effect on cancer multidrug resistance. *Mar Drugs.* 2012;10(10):2312-21.
[13] Fernandes J, Castilho RO, da Costa MR, Wagner-Souza K, Coelho Kaplan MA, Gattass CR. Pentacyclic triterpenes from Chrysobalanaceae species: cytotoxicity on multidrug resistant and sensitive leukemia cell lines. *Cancer Lett.* 2003;190(2):165-9.
[14] Madureira AM, Spengler G, Molnár A, Varga A, Molnár J, Abreu PM, et al. Effect of cycloartanes on reversal of multidrug resistance and apoptosis induction on mouse lymphoma cells. *Anticancer Res.* 2004;24(2B):859-64.
[15] Anreddy N, Gupta P, Kathawala RJ, Patel A, Wurpel JN, Chen ZS. Tyrosine kinase inhibitors as reversal agents for ABC transporter mediated drug resistance. *Molecules.* 2014;19(9):13848-77.
[16] Kathawala RJ, Gupta P, Ashby CR, Chen ZS. The modulation of ABC transporter-mediated multidrug resistance in cancer: a review of the past decade. *Drug Resist Updat.* 2015;18:1-17.
[17] Gupta P, Jani KA, Yang DH, Sadoqi M, Squillante E, Chen ZS. Revisiting the role of nanoparticles as modulators of drug resistance and metabolism in cancer. *Expert Opin Drug Metab Toxicol.* 2016;12(3):281-9.
[18] Krishna R, Mayer LD. Multidrug resistance (MDR) in cancer. Mechanisms, reversal using modulators of MDR and the role of MDR modulators in influencing the pharmacokinetics of anticancer drugs. *Eur J Pharm Sci.* 2000;11(4):265-83.
[19] Thomas H, Coley HM. Overcoming multidrug resistance in cancer: an update on the clinical strategy of inhibiting p-glycoprotein. *CancerControl.* 2003;10(2):159-65.
[20] Nobili S, Landini I, Giglioni B, Mini E. Pharmacological strategies for overcoming multidrug resistance. *Curr Drug Targets.* 2006;7(7):861-79.
[21] Zhang Y, Zhang YK, Wang YJ, Vispute SG, Jain S, Chen Y, et al. Esters of the marine-derived triterpene sipholenol A reverse P-GP-mediated drug resistance. *Mar Drugs.* 2015;13(4):2267-86.

[22] Jain S, Abraham I, Carvalho P, Kuang YH, Shaala LA, Youssef DT, et al. Sipholane triterpenoids: chemistry, reversal of ABCB1/P-glycoprotein-mediated multidrug resistance, and pharmacophore modeling. *J Nat Prod.* 2009;72(7):1291-8.

[23] Shi Z, Jain S, Kim IW, Peng XX, Abraham I, Youssef DT, et al. Sipholenol A, a marine-derived sipholane triterpene, potently reverses P-glycoprotein (ABCB1)-mediated multidrug resistance in cancer cells. *Cancer Sci.* 2007;98(9):1373-80.

[24] Liu DL, Li YJ, Yao N, Xu J, Chen ZS, Yiu A, et al. Acerinol, a cyclolanstane triterpenoid from Cimicifuga acerina, reverses ABCB1-mediated multidrug resistance in HepG2/ADM and MCF-7/ADR cells. *Eur J Pharmacol.* 2014;733:34-44.

[25] Nian Y, Zhu H, Tang WR, Luo Y, Du J, Qiu MH. Triterpenes from the aerial parts of Cimicifuga yunnanensis and their antiproliferative effects on p53(N236S) mouse embryonic fibroblasts. *J Nat Prod.* 2013;76(5):896-902.

[26] Kim SW, Kwon HY, Chi DW, Shim JH, Park JD, Lee YH, et al. Reversal of P-glycoprotein-mediated multidrug resistance by ginsenoside Rg(3). *Biochem Pharmacol.* 2003;65(1):75-82.

[27] Zhang DM, Shu C, Chen JJ, Sodani K, Wang J, Bhatnagar J, et al. BBA, a derivative of 23-hydroxybetulinic acid, potently reverses ABCB1-mediated drug resistance *in vitro* and *in vivo*. *Mol Pharm.* 2012;9(11):3147-59.

[28] Shan H, Qinglin Z, Fengjun X, Yuxin L, Xiaochen C, Yuan H. Reversal of multidrug resistance of KBV200 cells by triterpenoids isolated from Poria cocos. *Planta Med.* 2012;78(5):428-33.

[29] Yoshida N, Takada T, Yamamura Y, Adachi I, Suzuki H, Kawakami J. Inhibitory effects of terpenoids on multidrug resistance-associated protein 2- and breast cancer resistance protein-mediated transport. *DrugMetab Dispos.* 2008;36(7):1206-11.

[30] Zhang YK, Wang YJ, Gupta P, Chen ZS. Multidrug Resistance Proteins (MRPs) and Cancer Therapy. *AAPS J.* 2015.

[31] Braga F, Ayres-Saraiva D, Gattass CR, Capella MA. Oleanolic acid inhibits the activity of the multidrug resistance protein ABCC1 (MRP1) but not of the ABCB1 (P-glycoprotein): possible use in cancer chemotherapy. *Cancer Lett.* 2007;248(1):147-52.

[32] Hirrlinger J, König J, Keppler D, Lindenau J, Schulz JB, Dringen R. The multidrug resistance protein MRP1 mediates the release of glutathione disulfide from rat astrocytes during oxidative stress. *J Neurochem.* 2001;76(2):627-36.

In: Horizons in Cancer Research. Volume 63 ISBN: 978-1-53610-013-6
Editor: Hiroto S. Watanabe

Chapter 7

CANCER AND HEPARAN SULFATE ALTERATIONS

Iván Fernández-Vega[1], MD, PhD, Beatriz García[2], MD, PhD and Luis M. Quirós[2], MD, PhD

[1]Department of Pathology, Hospital Universitario de Araba-Txagorritxu, Spain

[2]Department of Functional Biology, University of Oviedo, 33006, Oviedo, Spain

ABSTRACT

Heparan sulfate proteoglycans (HSPGs) are glycoproteins, with the common characteristic of containing covalently attached heparan sulfate glycosaminoglycan chains (GAGs). GAGs have specific structural patterns generated through a series of interdependent enzymatic reactions that can involve various isoenzymes with differences in their specificities, responsible for the modification of the structure in physiological and pathological processes. In this light, HSPGS are highly modified in cancer, contributing to tumorigenesis. In fact, the expression of HSPGs is markedly altered during malignant transformation and tumor progression, affecting both the PG core proteins and the GAG chains. Numerous tumours show quantitative and structural alterations of heparan sulphate chains, largely caused by changes in the expression of the enzymes responsible for their biosynthesis, particularly at the fine structure level.

We discuss here some of the main regulatory points in HSPG formation and modification, all of which are implicated in cancer development and progression. Numerous tumours show quantitative and structural alterations largely caused by changes in the expression of the enzymes responsible for HSPGs biosynthesis, particularly at the fine structure level. The result is the alteration of the ligand binding sites responsible for directing specific cell signaling effects.

Cancer and Heparan Sulfate Alterations

Proteoglycans (PGs) are a diverse group of glycoconjugates composed of different core proteins covalently linked to linear chains of anionic polysaccharides called glycosaminoglycans (GAGs) which consist of repeating disaccharides. Heparan sulfate proteoglycans (HSPGs) comprise a specific small group of proteins with HS GAG chains. There are three known subfamilies of HSPGs: the glycophosphatidylinositol (GPI)-linked PGs called glypicans (GPCs); the membrane-spanning PGs known as syndecans (SDCs); and the secreted extracellular matrix (ECM) proteoglycans agrin, collagen XVIII and perlecan (PRCAN). Hematopoietic cells also contain a secretory vesicle proteoglycan called serglycin. Additionally, a few more proteins such as betaglycan and CD44v3 may appear as part-time HSPGs. In addition, some HSPGs can also have small proportions of chains of other types of GAGs attached to them [1].

HSPGs are structurally very complex, which means they possess large amounts of biological information, allowing them to participate in many different biological and pathological functions. This information is established by complex synthetic machinery encoded by around fifty different genes which are able to generate huge volumes of molecular combinations [2, 3]. Most of this biological information still remains unclear; however, the information contained in HS chains can develop precise biological roles and because of this many functions are attributed to both cell membrane and ECM HSPGs [4], including cell adhesion and migration, organization of the ECM, regulation of proliferation, differentiation and morphogenesis, cytoskeleton organization, tissue repair, inflammation, vascularization and cancer metastasis [4-6].

HS biosynthesis is not a random process, depending largely on transcriptional and translational controls that regulate the expression of the enzymes involved [7]. Furthermore, post-translational modifications of HSPGs can occur under the influence of other enzymes, especially extracellular sulfatases, heparanase (HPSE) and certain other sheddases [8].

The expression of HSPGs is markedly altered during malignant transformation and tumor progression, affecting both the PG core proteins and the GAG chains [9-12]. We show here the main enzymatic and regulatory alterations described in HSPG formation and modification, all of which are may well be involved in cancer development and progression. We highlight some examples of some of the alterations in the various steps of HSPG synthesis that give rise important changes in cell behavior and malignancy.

SYNTHESIS OF THE SACCHARIDIC CHAIN

The glycosyltransferases (GTs) involved in the biosynthesis of HS have been related with tumours. Thus, the genes *EXT1* and *EXT2* are tumour suppressors, associated with hereditary multiple exostoses [13, 14], characterized by the development of benign skeletal tumours in patients. It has also been suggested that the three *EXT*-like genes, *EXTL1-EXTL3*, may each be a tumour suppressor, although none is linked with HME [15]. There is less information concerning the synthesis of the linker although there are certain studies that have suggested a contribution of overexpression of GalT1 to cancer development and metastasis [16]. However, numerous studies show quantitative alterations in the absolute levels of HS and CS in different tumour processes [17, 18], which may be associated with alterations in expression levels of the GTs as in associated regulatory enzymes.

N-DEACETYLATION/N-SULPHATION

Despite the relevance of NDSTs in the generation of the sulphated domains in the HS structure, references in the literature to altered expression of NDSTs in tumours are scarce. However, some examples have been referred to such as the up-regulation of NDST-1 and NDST-2 in hepatocellular cancer [19] or the detection of NDST-4 transcripts in 50% of invasive breast ductal carcinomas [20]. An added difficulty in analysing the expression of these enzymes in tumours results from the fact that it has been described that the expression of the NDST isoforms may be both translationally and post-translationally regulated [21].

EPIMERIZATION

It has been suggested recently that epimerase is a relatively late evolutionary development and that its specificity, acting at an early point in the HS biosynthesis to convert GlcAGlcNS to IdoA-GlcNS in preference to converting GlcA-GlcNAc to IdoAGlcNAc, could constitute the basis for the relative abundance of these disaccharides [22]. However, there are few references to GlcA epimerase alterations in cancer although some data have been cited, such as significant down-regulation of its expression in human breast tumours, suggesting the genes possible involvement in carcinogenesis [23].

O-SULPHATION

During the biosynthetic process of the HS chains, different combinations of O-sulphate groups can be added to the C2 of uronic acid and to C6 and C3 of the glucosamine residues. There is some evidence that 2-O-sulphotransferase (2-OST) can be associated with tumour progression. This is the case in prostate cancer where it is overexpressed in tumours and cell lines; 2-OST is essential for proliferation and invasion, and its expression correlates with increasing metastatic potential. It has also been suggested that up-regulation of 2-OST expression could produce a more efficient form of highly sulphated perlecan in metastatic prostate cancer tumours that fail to show increase in perlecan protein levels [24].

In Addition, there are three forms of 6-O-sulphotransferases, 6-OST-1-3, which show differences in their substrate specificities and tissue expression [21]. Alterations in the expression levels of one or more of these isoforms have been referenced in different tumours. Furthermore, strong expression of 6-OST-1 and overexpression of 6-OST-2 have been described in ovarian cancer although the HS molecules produced subsequently act as substrate for extracellular enzymes which modulate their biological function [25]. Up-regulation of 6-OST-2 has also been mentioned in relation to human colorectal cancers in conjunction with alterations in the expression levels of some syndecans, while the predominant form present in normal mucous is 6-OST-3 [17]. Moreover, 6-OST-1 is upregulated in hepatocellular cancer although the overexpression of extracellular sulphatases resolves in modest 6-O-undersulphation of HS [19]. However, in other tumour types subexpression of these enzymes has been described; thus, 6-OST-1-3 are down-regulated in glioblastoma, although the alterations in the expression of some PGs and HS biosynthetic enzymes in these tumours is altered in a subtype-specific manner [26]. The last family of enzymes that are involved in the modification of HS are the 3-O-sulphotransferases. Numerous studies have described alterations of these proteins in different tumours. Some up-regulations have been reported, as is the case of 3-OST-1 or 3-OST-3A in hepatocellular cancer, glioblastoma and breast cancer, respectively [19, 26, 27]. However, in many cases sub-expressions of different isoforms have been determined; methylation-associated silencing of 3-OST-2 has been described in breast, colon, lung and pancreatic cancers [28], and in human malignant melanoma [29]. Hypermethylation of 3-OST-2, as well as 3-OST-1 and 3-OST-3A, appears in chondrosarcoma cells, contributing to the invasive phenotype [30]. Furthermore, down-regulation of isoforms 3-OST-4, 3-OST-5 and 3-OST-6 have been described in invasive breast ductal carcinomas [20].

EXTRACELLULAR ENDOSULPHATASES

There are many reported data that describe alterations in the expression of these enzymes in cancer: Sulf-2 is up-regulated in various tumours such as glioblastoma, breast, hepatocellular or pancreatic carcinoma [17, 19, 20, 26]. Sulf-1 has been described as up-regulated in some tumours such as glioblastoma, ovarian, breast, hepatocellular or pancreatic carcinoma [19, 20, 25, 28, 31], while other reports indicate a down-regulation in ovarian, head and neck, breast or hepatocellular carcinomas [17, 32]. The existence of alternative splicing variants of these enzymes has been described and related to divergences in expression in some tumours [33].

FRAGMENTATION OF HEPARAN SULFATE CHAINS BY HEPARANASE

HPSE is an endo-β-D-glucuronidase that is capable of cleaving HS side chains of HSPGs on cell surfaces and the ECM, an activity that is strongly implicated in cancer progression, invasion and tumor metastasis. The HPSE releases fragments that are biologically active [34], influencing the activity and availability of numerous HS-binding factors that regulate cell behavior of both the tumor cells and host cells within the tumor microenvironment [8].

SHEDDING OF PROTEOGLYCAN EXTRACELLULAR DOMAINS

SDCs are, up to the present time, the best studied HSPGs with many cases of increased shedding having been reported in these proteoglycans in cancer. Many sheddases (matrix metalloproteinases) have been described which participate in this process and it can have a dramatic impact on cell behavior, especially on cell adhesion and the formation of growth factor gradients, which is extremely important for cancer progression [35].

Matrix metalloproteinases are able to release intact syndecan ectodomains from the cell surface giving rise to a soluble, shed form of the PG. The shed form of SDC can facilitate the growth, angiogenesis, and metastasis of tumors, playing an active role in the tumoral niche and serum. In fact, studies have demonstrated that high levels of serum SDC1 are an indicator of poor prognosis in both myeloma and lung cancer, and associated with increased growth and metastasis [36]. Moreover, stromal expression of SDC1 in pancreatic cancer is correlated with worse outcomes, as well as being an independent prognostic factor. On the contrary, stromal expression of SDC2 has no significant influence on the prognosis of pancreatic cancer, while epithelial expression is strongly correlated with better outcomes. This fact confirms that in cancer epithelial and stromal SDCs have different functions and that these are related to their locations [37].

Finally, HSPGs show a highly modified structure in many cancers, through abnormalities at either the transcriptional, translational or post-translational level. Several examples endorse the fact that these molecules play an important role in carcinogenesis and tumor progression. However, understanding the biosynthetic regulation of HSPGs and decoding the heparanome remain a challenge for scientists in order to fully comprehend the whole process, that is to say, the main functions that HSPGs might actually play in cancer. Once we are able to unravel these as yet unclear roles of HSPGs in cancer, a gate might be opened toward the creation of new anti-cancer drugs.

REFERENCES

[1] Bishop JR, Schuksz M, Esko JD. Heparan sulphate proteoglycans fine-tune mammalian physiology. *Nature.* 2007 Apr 26;446 (7139): 1030-7.
[2] Lamanna WC, Kalus I, Padva M, Baldwin RJ, Merry CL, Dierks T. The heparanome--the enigma of encoding and decoding heparan sulfate sulfation. *J. Biotechnol.* 2007 Apr 30;129 (2): 290-307.
[3] Zhang X, Wang F, Sheng J. "Coding" and "Decoding": hypothesis for the regulatory mechanism involved in heparan sulfate biosynthesis. *Carbohydr. Res.* 2016 Apr 8;428: 1-7.
[4] Ori A, Wilkinson MC, Fernig DG. The heparanome and regulation of cell function: structures, functions and challenges. *Front Biosci.* 2008;13: 4309-38.
[5] Suhovskih AV, Domanitskaya NV, Tsidulko AY, Prudnikova TY, Kashuba VI, Grigorieva EV. Tissue-specificity of heparan sulfate biosynthetic machinery in cancer. *Cell Adh. Migr.* 2015;9 (6): 452-9.
[6] Knelson EH, Nee JC, Blobe GC. Heparan sulfate signaling in cancer. *Trends Biochem. Sci.* 2014 Jun;39 (6): 277-88.
[7] Kreuger J, Kjellen L. Heparan sulfate biosynthesis: regulation and variability. *J. Histochem. Cytochem.* 2012 Dec;60 (12): 898-907.
[8] Sanderson RD, Yang Y, Kelly T, MacLeod V, Dai Y, Theus A. Enzymatic remodeling of heparan sulfate proteoglycans within the tumor microenvironment: growth regulation and the prospect of new cancer therapies. *J. Cell Biochem.* 2005 Dec 1;96 (5): 897-905.
[9] García-Suárez O F-VI, Quirós LM. Multiple alterations of heparan sulphate in cancer. *OA Cancer.* [Review]. 2013;01 (1): 1.
[10] Fernández-Vega I GB, García-Suarez O, Castañon S, Quirós LM. Alterations of Heparan Sulfate Proteoglycans in Cancer. *Journal of Glycobiology.* 2014;3 (109).
[11] García-Suárez O Fernandez-Vega I QL. Multiple alterations of heparan sulphate in cancer. *OA Cancer.* 2013;1(1).

[12] Fernandez-Vega I, Garcia-Suarez O, Garcia B, Crespo A, Astudillo A, Quiros LM. Heparan sulfate proteoglycans undergo differential expression alterations in right sided colorectal cancer, depending on their metastatic character. *BMC Cancer.* 2015;15: 742.

[13] Hartmann G, Prospero T, Brinkmann V, Ozcelik C, Winter G, Hepple J, et al. Engineered mutants of HGF/SF with reduced binding to heparan sulphate proteoglycans, decreased clearance and enhanced activity in vivo. *Curr. Biol.* 1998 Jan 29;8 (3): 125-34.

[14] Iozzo RV, Sanderson RD. Proteoglycans in cancer biology, tumour microenvironment and angiogenesis. *J. Cell Mol. Med.* 2011 May;15 (5): 1013-31.

[15] Nadanaka S, Zhou S, Kagiyama S, Shoji N, Sugahara K, Sugihara K, et al. EXTL2, a member of the EXT family of tumor suppressors, controls glycosaminoglycan biosynthesis in a xylose kinase-dependent manner. *J. Biol. Chem.* 2013 Mar 29;288 (13): 9321-33.

[16] Bret C, Hose D, Reme T, Sprynski AC, Mahtouk K, Schved JF, et al. Expression of genes encoding for proteins involved in heparan sulphate and chondroitin sulphate chain synthesis and modification in normal and malignant plasma cells. *Br. J. Haematol.* 2009 May;145 (3): 350-68.

[17] Raman K, Kuberan B. Chemical Tumor Biology of Heparan Sulfate Proteoglycans. *Curr. Chem. Biol.* 2010 Jan 1;4 (1): 20-31.

[18] Batista LT, Matos LL, Machado LR, Suarez ER, Theodoro TR, Martins JR, et al. Heparanase expression and glycosaminoglycans profile in renal cell carcinoma. *Int. J. Urol.* 2012 Nov;19 (11): 1036-40.

[19] Tatrai P, Egedi K, Somoracz A, van Kuppevelt TH, Ten Dam G, Lyon M, et al. Quantitative and qualitative alterations of heparan sulfate in fibrogenic liver diseases and hepatocellular cancer. *J. Histochem. Cytochem.* 2010 May;58 (5): 429-41.

[20] Fernandez-Vega I, Garcia O, Crespo A, Castanon S, Menendez P, Astudillo A, et al. Specific genes involved in synthesis and editing of heparan sulfate proteoglycans show altered expression patterns in breast cancer. *BMC Cancer.* 2013;13: 24.

[21] Esko JD, Selleck SB. Order out of chaos: assembly of ligand binding sites in heparan sulfate. *Annu. Rev. Biochem.* 2002;71: 435-71.

[22] Rudd TR, Yates EA. A highly efficient tree structure for the biosynthesis of heparan sulfate accounts for the commonly observed disaccharides and suggests a mechanism for domain synthesis. *Mol. Biosyst.* 2012 Apr;8 (5): 1499-506.

[23] Grigorieva EV, Prudnikova TY, Domanitskaya NV, Mostovich LA, Pavlova TV, Kashuba VI, et al. D-glucuronyl C5-epimerase suppresses small-cell lung cancer cell proliferation in vitro and tumour growth in vivo. *Br. J. Cancer.* 2011 Jun 28;105 (1): 74-82.

[24] Ferguson BW DS. Role of heparan sulphate 2-O-sulfotransferase in prostate cancer cell proliferation, invasion and growth factor signalling. *Prostate Cancer.* 2011.

[25] Backen AC, Cole CL, Lau SC, Clamp AR, McVey R, Gallagher JT, et al. Heparan sulphate synthetic and editing enzymes in ovarian cancer. *Br. J. Cancer.* 2007 May 21;96 (10): 1544-8.

[26] Wade A, Robinson AE, Engler JR, Petritsch C, James CD, Phillips JJ. Proteoglycans and their roles in brain cancer. *FEBS J.* 2013 May;280 (10): 2399-417.

[27] Mao X, Gauche C, Coughtrie MW, Bui C, Gulberti S, Merhi-Soussi F, et al. The heparan sulfate sulfotransferase 3-OST3A (HS3ST3A) is a novel tumor regulator and a prognostic marker in breast cancer. *Oncogene.* 2016 Apr 4.

[28] Miyamoto K, Asada K, Fukutomi T, Okochi E, Yagi Y, Hasegawa T, et al. Methylation-associated silencing of heparan sulfate D-glucosaminyl 3-O-sulfotransferase-2 (3-OST-2) in human breast, colon, lung and pancreatic cancers. *Oncogene.* 2003 Jan 16;22 (2): 274-80.

[29] Furuta J, Umebayashi Y, Miyamoto K, Kikuchi K, Otsuka F, Sugimura T, et al. Promoter methylation profiling of 30 genes in human malignant melanoma. *Cancer Sci.* 2004 Dec;95 (12): 962-8.

[30] Bui C, Ouzzine M, Talhaoui I, Sharp S, Prydz K, Coughtrie MW, et al. Epigenetics: methylation-associated repression of heparan sulfate 3-O-sulfotransferase gene expression contributes to the invasive phenotype of H-EMC-SS chondrosarcoma cells. *FASEB J.* 2010 Feb;24 (2): 436-50.

[31] Nawroth R, van Zante A, Cervantes S, McManus M, Hebrok M, Rosen SD. Extracellular sulfatases, elements of the Wnt signaling pathway, positively regulate growth and tumorigenicity of human pancreatic cancer cells. *PLoS One.* 2007;2 (4): e392.

[32] Narita K, Staub J, Chien J, Meyer K, Bauer M, Friedl A, et al. HSulf-1 inhibits angiogenesis and tumorigenesis in vivo. *Cancer Res.* 2006 Jun 15;66 (12): 6025-32.

[33] Gill RB, Day A, Barstow A, Zaman G, Chenu C, Dhoot GK. Mammalian Sulf1 RNA alternative splicing and its significance to tumour growth regulation. *Tumour Biol.* 2012 Oct;33 (5): 1669-80.

[34] Bitan M, Polliack A, Zecchina G, Nagler A, Friedmann Y, Nadav L, et al. Heparanase expression in human leukemias is restricted to acute myeloid leukemias. *Exp. Hematol.* 2002 Jan;30 (1): 34-41.

[35] Fitzgerald ML, Wang Z, Park PW, Murphy G, Bernfield M. Shedding of syndecan-1 and -4 ectodomains is regulated by multiple signaling pathways and mediated by a TIMP-3-sensitive metalloproteinase. *J. Cell Biol.* 2000 Feb 21;148 (4): 811-24.

[36] Dhodapkar MV, Kelly T, Theus A, Athota AB, Barlogie B, Sanderson RD. Elevated levels of shed syndecan-1 correlate with tumour mass and decreased matrix metalloproteinase-9 activity in the serum of patients with multiple myeloma. *Br. J. Haematol.* 1997 Nov;99 (2): 368-71.

[37] Hrabar D, Aralica G, Gomercic M, Ljubicic N, Kruslin B, Tomas D. Epithelial and stromal expression of syndecan-2 in pancreatic carcinoma. *Anticancer Res.* 2010 Jul;30 (7): 2749-53.

In: Horizons in Cancer Research. Volume 63 ISBN: 978-1-53610-013-6
Editor: Hiroto S. Watanabe

Chapter 8

GANODERMA LUCIDUM TARGETING APOPTOSIS: BOON TO MANKIND

Balraj Singh Gill, Navgeet and Sanjeev Kumar*
Centre for Biosciences, School of Basic and Applied Sciences,
Central University of Punjab, Bathinda, India

ABSTRACT

Cancer is a multifactorial disease involving network of genes, controlling the functions of the cell. Use of sophisticated tool and techniques in molecular biology revealed the mechanistic binding of numerous genes indulged in the progression of cancer. A wide range of synthetic products was synthesized; whose efficiency decreased the mortality rate from last few decades. Natural products serve as templates to synthesize new efficient products in the cancer treatment. A broad spectrum of antibiotics and drugs were obtained from natural products without any detrimental effect. Among natural products, terpenes emerged as a better class in modulating various signaling pathway in cancer. In cancer, topoisomerases play a crucial role in controlling replication, transcription, and translation process. Topoisomerases regulates the overwinding or underwinding of DNA which regulates the functioning of cell cycle. One of the renowned medicinal mushrooms,

* Corresponding Author, Centre for Biosciences, School of Basic and Applied Sciences, Central University of Punjab, Bathinda-151001 India. E-mail: sanjeevpuchd@gmail.com, sanjeevcbs@cup.ac.in. Tel: + 91 9501278687.

Ganoderma lucidum targets various pathways in cancer, one among them is apoptosis. Ganoderic acid, triterpenes isolated from *Ganoderma lucidum*, played crucial role in apoptosis pathway were studied in this chapter.

Keywords: *Ganoderma lucidum,* ganoderic acid, topoisomerases, cancer, terpenes

INTRODUCTION

Cancer is marked by multifactorial complex events in progression and development which makethe cancer invasive and aggressive [1]. Cancer is primarily caused by somatic mutations, whereas others result from mutations in the germline [2]. Alteration or the mutation in the critical genes, epigenetic silencing, and disorganization in the function of the cell, causes cancer. The activation of the proteins is regulated or controlled by switching on or off of membrane receptors which get phosphorylated and activate proteins for signaling in the progression of cancer. Failure of the complex network involved in signaling cascade consequence in cancer progression and difficult for the researcher to target a particular protein responsible for causing cancer.1,685,210 new cases of cancer have been reported in this year alone, of which595,690 deaths have been reported in the United States alone. The reports explicit the variation in a number of cancer patients related with particular sex. Though cancer mortality among men has been reduced by 3.1% as compared to 2009-2012 population statistics, cancer mortality among females still remains unchanged, thus highlighting the dependence of cancer on gender specific genes providing researchers the platform to work in this direction [3]. Nature provides the variety of medicinal plants, which target the signaling in the cancer through the process of apoptosis. Broad ranges of drugs were synthesized by using either pure natural compounds or acts as template to synthesize other products. Some of the products of natural compounds have passed FDA approval, whereas some are still in dark and need focus to highlight their medicinal efficacy [4]. Advancement and use of modern techniques has yielded new drug formulation helpful in reducing mortality [5, 6]. Natural products or semi-synthetic compounds inhibit the development of dreadful diseases by blocking or reversing the process in the signaling. The bioactive compounds present in natural products engraved with antioxidants, phenolics and capacity to inhibit free radicals makes them pivotal therapeutics.

Natural products have contributed towards numerous drugs such as paclitaxel, vinblastine, and vincristine indicated in HIV/AIDS, Alzheimer's disease, malaria and cancer [7]. Thus, provides an edge with new structural leads for effective drug development [8].

Among natural products, terpenes are the major class of natural products with immense power to combat cosmopolitan diseases such as cancer. Terpenes are biosynthetically produced from the basic units known as isoprene. The categorization and properties exhibited by terpenoids divided into subclasses and their activity vary from anti-inflammatory, antitumorigenic, and hypolipidemic activity [9]. Structurally, triterpenes are categorized into different forms based on number of isoprene units as monoterpenes (C_{10}), sesquiterpenes (C_{15}), diterpenes (C_{20}), sesquiterpenes (C_{25}), triterpenes (C_{30}), and tetraterpenes (C_{40}), where the carbon skeleton is cyclic, or contains mono, bi, tri, tetra, and pentacyclic structures respectively. As terpenes as part of secondary metabolism, which are derived from C5 isoprene units joints in a head-to-tail fashion.

Triterpenes are produced as a result of the arrangement of squalene epoxide in a chair-chair-chair-boat arrangement [10]. Triterpenes forms important structural components in plant membranes and plays a critical role in the stability of cell membrane [10]. The basic unit of terpenoids biosynthesisis known as isoprene, which has isopentenyl pyrophosphate (IPP) and its isomer dimethyl allyl pyrophosphate (DMAPP) available in its activate form the basis for the synthesis of terpenoids [9]. Acetyl-CoA forms the basis of IPP formation via intermediate formation of mevalonic acid in the HMG-CoA reductase (HMGR) pathway. In addition, the process of cyclizations of three prenyltransferasessynthesizesprenyl pyrophosphates, geranyl pyrophosphate (GPP), farnesyl pyrophosphate (FPP), and geranylgeranyl pyrophosphate (GGPP) [11].

Topoisomerase is a class of enzyme critically involved in the process of duplication, transcription, translation, and cellular transactions. During breakage reaction of the DNA strand, tyrosyl oxygen of topoisomerase enzyme attack phosphorous, forming phosphotyrosine link which results in the breakage of a phosphodiester bond. Rejoining occurs by transesterification and creates transient enzyme-mediated gates in the DNA [12]. DNA topoisomerase includes two categories - type I and type II. Type I is a 91 kDa monomeric unit, relax both positive and negative supercoil and break only one strand. Type II is 174kDa exists in homodimeric form and cut both strands of the double helix and then reanneals the cut strand. A wide spectrum of antibiotics is based on the activity of topoisomerases, effectively targeting DNA replication, particularly bacterial gyrase (topoisomerase II and topoisomerase IV) against numerous diseases [12].

One of the important basidiomycete fungi which remain in dark since a long time, known as *Ganoderma lucidum* (*G. lucidum*), used as herbal medicine. Locally known as *Reishi* or *lingZhi* in China and Japan respectively, and their morphology depends on the geographical origin and host-specific interdependence on plant [13]. Different species of *Ganoderma lucidum* characterized by their morphological and anatomical features, such as shape and size of the basidiocarp, the color of pileus, stipe, and pore size [14]. Different ethanol, methanol, acetone, chloroform, ether, water extract of *Ganoderma lucidum* ranges in the medicinal property causing activation of different pathway in cancer. *G. lucidum* contains a wide variety of bioactive constituents such as terpenoids, steroids, phenols, glycoprotein, and polysaccharides. Among terpenoids, ganoderic acid forms major class with more than 100 isoforms. The basic lanosterol moiety remains the same, whereas functional groups change and thus modulates the functioning of the particular isoform. Ganoderic acid acts as a key player among terpenes with multiple roles in signaling pathway [15].

GANODERMA AND TOPOISOMERASES

A mixture of methanolic and aqueous extract of fruiting and spores of *Ganoderma lucidum* exhibits inhibitory action on tumor cells and DNA topoisomerases [16]. Lanostanoid triterpene ganoderic acid X (GA-X) isolated from *Ganoderma amboinense* inhibits topoisomerases and modulates the signaling in the process of apoptosis. GA-X inhibits DNA synthesis by activating cell apoptosis by modulating signaling of ERK and JNK mitogen-activated protein kinases. GA-X hampers the mitochondrial membrane potential, Bcl, cytochrome c and the functioning of caspases. Thus, study concludes that GA-X target topoisomerases and different protein controlling the process of apoptosis, and emerge as a therapeutic tool in apoptosis [17]. Similarly, ganoderic acid T (GA-T) inhibit the activity of topoisomerases in a dose-dependent manner by interfering by forming complex formation by formation of competitive inhibition by the substitute [18]. Triterpenes ganoderiol F (GolF), isolated from *Ganoderma amboinense,* found to induce senescence and exhibits anticancer potential. GolF inhibits the activity of topoisomerase, and therefore inhibits the synthesis of cellular DNA. Effect of

GolF activates EKR signaling and leads to the up-regulation of cyclin-dependent kinase inhibitor in the HepG2 cells [19].

GANODERMA IN PROCESS OF APOPTOSIS

Ganoderma regulates the functioning of the cell and, if the process of apoptosis goes awry, results in progression of cancer [20]. *Ganoderma* modulates the expression level of different protein by upregulating or downregulating of adapter molecules in a signaling cascade initiated by membrane receptors. The unique morphology and biochemical changes in the cell functioning lead to initiate apoptosis, and any deregulation in the process result in cancer [21]. The process of apoptosis acts either in intrinsic or extrinsic pathways, in which intrinsic pathways is targeted by an anti-apoptotic and pro-apoptotic factor of Bcl-2. Ganoderic acid DM (GA-DM) increases the expression of bax protein, Apaf-1, cytochrome-c, Beclin-1, and LC3 proteins resulting in the process of apoptosis. GA-DM stimulates the autophagy and enhances the immunity against cancer cells [22]. Ganoderic acid Mf (GA-Mf) and ganoderic acid S (GA-S) isolated from mycelia of *Ganoderma lucidum* induces the process of cell apoptosis in HeLa cells. Treatment of both isoforms of ganoderic acid varies in causing impact in different cell cycle stages. GA-S exhibits more potential in S phase of cell cycle, whereas GA-Mf acts efficiently on G1 phase. Both isomers of ganoderic acid decrease the mitochondrial membrane potential which consequences in the release of cytochrome c from the cytosol and changes the mitochondrial potential. This change causes alteration in Bax/Bcl-2 ratio giving the way to apoptosis in HeLa cells [23].

Ganoderic acid Me (GA-Me) induced p53-mediated G1 arrest and induce apoptosis in the human colon cells. GA-Me treatment causes decreases in overall ratio of Bcl-2/Bax, with upregulation of Bax, without changing the expression of Bcl-2. GA-Me decreases the mitochondrial membrane potential with participation of caspases and cytochrome c and induced the process of apoptosis in human colon carcinoma cells [24]. Ganoderic acid T (GA-T), isolated from a methanolic extract of *Ganoderma lucidum,* suppress the growth of tumor in athymic mice. GA-T arrests the G1 phase of cell cycle and inhibits the proliferation of a highly metastatic lung cancer. GA-T results in intrinsic mitochondrial-mediated apoptosis and can be potentially useful as chemotherapeutic agent [25].

CONCLUSION

Topoisomerases control the functioning of the cells by controlling the DNA replication. Terpenes have emerged as a new class with different subclasses hampering the cellular cascading responsible for numerous dreadful diseases in cancer. Medicinal mushroom proves their impact in handling cancer to some extent. Medicinal mushrooms are being used since ancient time without knowing their medicinal effect thus making scientific community curious to isolate compounds to target in cancer. Among various isolated compounds, ganoderic acid originates in various isoforms with medicinal potential. Ganoderic acid is potentially known for the anticancerous property, interfering the process of topoisomerase. Along with the replication process, some of the alcoholic products of *Ganoderma* interfere in cell cycle regulation. Natural products and its products provide the templates to synthesize such compounds which target topoisomerases. Different isoforms of ganoderic acid share basic lanostane moiety, which varies in the functional group. The functioning of different isoforms provides the edge and clue to the researcher about the selectivity of the side chain in a particular protein. The present group is engaged in determining the anticancer property of *Ganoderma lucidum* and its bioactive compounds. The present group performed the chemical profiling of *Ganoderma lucidum* in the stress condition and interdependency of *Ganoderma lucidum* with the different host-specific plant. Along with this, the group also demonstrates how ganoderic acids activate different receptor tyrosine kinase in cancer signaling.

ACKNOWLEDGMENT

BSG, NG, SK thank Central University of Punjab, Bathinda for providing the necessary facilities to carry out the present work. The authors acknowledge and thank Jimi Marin Alex for assistance in editing the article. Balraj Singh Gill thanks UGC for Maulana Azad National fellowship (F1-17.1/2011-12/MANF-SIK-HIM-3205).

Conflict of Interest

None.

REFERENCES

[1] Gill B, Alex J, Kumar S. Missing link between microRNA and prostate cancer. *Tumour biology: the journal of the International Society for Oncodevelopmental Biology and Medicine*. 2016;37(5):5683-704.

[2] Anand SS, Gill BS. Breakthroughs in epigenetics. *PharmaTutor*. 2015; 3(7):16-24.

[3] Siegel RL, Miller KD, Jemal A. Cancer statistics, 2016. *CA: a cancer journal for clinicians*. 2016;66(1):7-30.

[4] Newman DJ, Cragg GM. Natural Products as Sources of New Drugs over the Last 25 Years. *Journal of natural products*. 2007;70(3):461-77.

[5] A Negi BG, SS Anand. Tilling: Versatile Reverse Genetic Tool. *PharmaTutor*. 2014;2(1):26-32.

[6] Negi A, Gill B. Success stories of enolate form of drugs. *PharmaTutor*. 2013;1(2):45-53.

[7] Yin M-C. Anti-glycative potential of triterpenes: a mini-review. *BioMedicine*. 2012;2(1):2-9.

[8] Cragg GM, Newman DJ. Natural products: a continuing source of novel drug leads. *Biochimica et Biophysica Acta (BBA)-General Subjects*. 2013;1830(6):3670-95.

[9] Gill BS, Kumar S, Navgeet. Triterpenes in cancer: significance and their influence. *Molecular Biology Reports*. 2016:1-16. doi:10.1007/s11033-016-4032-9.

[10] Liby KT, Yore MM, Sporn MB. Triterpenoids and rexinoids as multifunctional agents for the prevention and treatment of cancer. *Nature Reviews Cancer*. 2007;7(5):357-69.

[11] Liang PH, Ko TP, Wang AHJ. Structure, mechanism and function of prenyltransferases. *European Journal of Biochemistry*. 2002;269(14): 3339-54.

[12] Liu LF. DNA topoisomerase poisons as antitumor drugs. *Annual review of biochemistry*. 1989;58(1):351-75.

[13] Gill BS, Sharma P, Kumar R, Kumar S. Misconstrued versatility of *Ganoderma lucidum*: a key player in multi-targeted cellular signaling. *Tumor Biology*. 2016;37(3):2789-804.

[14] Bhosle S, Ranadive K, Bapat G, Garad S, Deshpande G, Vaidya J. Taxonomy and diversity of Ganoderma from the Western parts of Maharashtra (India). *Mycosphere*. 2010;1(3):249-62.

[15] Gill BS, Kumar S. Differential algorithms-assisted molecular modeling-based identification of mechanistic binding of ganoderic acids. *Medicinal Chemistry Research*. 2015;24(9):3483-93.

[16] Chun C, Hengbang W, Yingying W, Jianhua X, Ye L, Zhiyong X. Inhibitory effects of *Ganoderma lucidum* extracts and spores oil on tumor cells *in vitro* and *in vivo* and on DNA topoisomerases [J]. *Pharmacology and Clinics of Chinese Materia Medica*. 2008;2:022.

[17] Li C-H, Chen P-Y, Chang U-M, Kan L-S, Fang W-H, Tsai K-S et al. Ganoderic acid X, a lanostanoid triterpene, inhibits topoisomerases and induces apoptosis of cancer cells. *Life sciences*. 2005;77(3):252-65.

[18] Wen T. The Inhibition Effect of Triterpenoid in Ganoderma on Topoisomerase. *Journal of Shanghai Institute of Technology (Natural Science)*. 2011;2:001.

[19] Chang U-M, Li C-H, Lin L-I, Huang C-P, Kan L-S, Lin S-B. Ganoderiol F, a ganoderma triterpene, induces senescence in hepatoma HepG2 cells. *Life sciences*. 2006;79(12):1129-39.

[20] Gill BS KS. Homology Model of Galu_Mp19: LAGLIDADG. British *Journal of Medical and Health Research*. 2014;2(1).

[21] Shivakumar SB, Bharti D, Subbarao RB, Jang SJ, Park JS, Ullah I et al. DMSO-and Serum-Free Cryopreservation of Wharton's Jelly Tissue Isolated from Human Umbilical Cord. *Journal of Cellular Biochemistry*. 2016.

[22] Wu G-S, Lu J-J, Guo J-J, Li Y-B, Tan W, Dang Y-Y et al. Ganoderic acid DM, a natural triterpenoid, induces DNA damage, G1 cell cycle arrest and apoptosis in human breast cancer cells. *Fitoterapia*. 2012; 83(2):408-14.

[23] Liu R-M, Zhong J-J. Ganoderic acid Mf and S induce mitochondria mediated apoptosis in human cervical carcinoma HeLa cells. *Phytomedicine*. 2011;18(5):349-55.

[24] Zhou L, Shi P, Chen N-H, Zhong J-J. Ganoderic acid Me induces apoptosis through mitochondria dysfunctions in human colon carcinoma cells. *Process Biochemistry*. 2011;46(1):219-25.

[25] Tang W, Liu J-W, Zhao W-M, Wei D-Z, Zhong J-J. Ganoderic acid T from *Ganoderma lucidum* mycelia induces mitochondria mediated apoptosis in lung cancer cells. *Life sciences*. 2006;80(3):205-11.

In: Horizons in Cancer Research. Volume 63 ISBN: 978-1-53610-013-6
Editor: Hiroto S. Watanabe

Chapter 9

The Integrated Model of cAMP-Dependent DNA Expression Reveals an Inverse Relationship Between Cancer and Neurodegeneration

Alfred Bennun, PhD
Full Professor-Emeritus, Rutgers University, US

Abstract

The model for cAMP-dependent synaptic plasticity relates the characterization of a noradrenaline-stimulated adenylyl cyclase with DNA unzipping. Specific proteins condition cAMP insertion in specific sites of the DNA structure to direct cellular and synaptic differentiation in brain tissues, also providing coding. Metabolic-dependent ATP binding of Mg^{2+}, could control feedback by inactivating AC dependent formation of cAMP. The level of cAMP and cGMP, which could be assayed in red cells and cerebrospinal fluid, allows a clinical lab diagnostic improvement. Also, provides a relationship of best fitting to cAMP control by binding to DNA. The cAMP level allows the prediction of an inverse relationship between neurodegeneration and cancer. The latter, could be characterized by uncontrolled proliferation, whereas metabolic dominance by stress over a long period of time, may deplete cerebral cAMP.

INTRODUCTION

The study of noradrenaline (NA)-stimulated adenylyl cyclase (AC) [EC 4.6.1.1] of rat brain hypothalamus, cortex and corpus striatum [1], indicated a requirement for an excess of Mg^{2+} over substrate MgATP. Mg^{2+}-ion at far greater concentrations resulted in basal activation curve of basal AC, but at considerable greater Mg^{2+} excess over substrate.

DNA by heating at about 65°C results in uncoiling of its helix structure separating its two strands structure. The AC product, cAMP in conjunction with Me^{2+} (Mg^{2+}, Zn^{2+}, Mn^{2+}) has a similar capacity for opening the structure of DNA [2]. Accordingly the tendency to form DNA-Me^{2+}-cAMP complexes uncoils a DNA segment, forming with the now separated strands a triple-stranded structure. Characterization as an epigenetic mechanism results from the ATP capacity to chelate the ligand metal, releasing cAMP from the complex.

This one allows to predict mechanisms for a role of cAMP on DNA unzipping and transcription. The red cell without mitochondria and DNA controls the Pasteur Effect. This one shows that an O_2-dependent increase of citric cycle activity at the mitochondrial inhibits glycolysis at the cytoplasmic level.

The cAMP-ERK1/2-Bad signaling pathways by toxic levels of 6-OHDA (6-hydroxydopamine) a role in dopamine neuronal death of animal models for Parkinson's disease [3].

Uncontrolled cell division in cancer, circumvent apoptotic pathways, the patients show lower risk for neurodegenerative diseases, involving neuronal apoptosis, like Parkinson and Alzheimer [4]. This reverse relationship suggests sharing of a similar mechanism with different outcomes.

The reverse metabolic relationship characterizes cancer in many tissues. The Mg^{2+} chelating capacity of ATP modulates the Mg^{2+}-dependent activity of adrenaline-stimulated AC [5] [6].

The nucleotide cAMP and cGMP bind DNA in a rather non-reversible and stable coding except in the presence of a stronger, chelating agent like ATP^{4-}.

This provides a metabolic connection for the cAMP level control of DNA expression, which at the brain could individualize neurons implicating the receptors proteins. Thus, allowing synaptic plasticity to function as memory networks.

RESULTS

Similarly, cAMP has been reported involved in CREB (cAMP response element-binding), protein that is involved as factor transcription and which is a part of memory function for many laboratories. This finding resulted in the development of behavior-cAMP linked models [2] [7] [8] [9] [10] [11] [12].

Kosmotropic (order-making) versus chaotropic (order-breaking) co-solvents influence equilibrium in aqueous solutions of proteins, acting through the structure and dynamics of the hydration water surrounding a protein [13]. The double hydration shell of $Mg^{2+}/Zn^{2+}/Me^{2+}$ allows conformational changes to enzymes and proteins, like hemoglobin. The turnover depends of an Mg^{2+} binding to a protein requires losses on the hydration shell to form a chelate. This may have the tendency to decrease its hydration water and increasing the effective charge *nascent* ions like Mg^{2+} could also explain Zn^{2+}/Mn^{2+}-fingers. Lately other groups provided a more fashionable denomination as Zn^{2+} fingers, the chemistry is the same [14] [15] [16]. A divalent metal when attracted by more than one negative group constitutes a chelated state.

Mg^{2+} when released by proteins like oxyHb turnover into deoxyHb appears in *nascent* state seeking water from the hydration shell of other ions like Na^+ and K^+.

These tendencies adjust the size of the hydration shells of Na^+ and K^+ ions for fitting into the gate-dynamics of the Na^+-ion-pump.

The chaotropic strength could capture H_2O from the kosmotropic $[K(H_2O)_6]^+$ to generate tetra-hydrated $[K(H_2O)_4]^+$ and tri-hydrated complexes $[K(H_2O)_3]^+$.

OxyHb regenerative effect on tissues at lower pH appears to depend on the release by red cells of O_2, Mg^{2+} and cAMP/cGMP. The latter ones provide the DNA unzipping effect involved in transcription to generate the require polypeptides and proteins. In brain this coding effect creates memory at the level of individual neurons which function in neuronal networks [3].

This structure is reversible by the releasing of the ion Mg^{2+} by a negative charged molecule with great affinity for Mg^{2+} like ATP^{4-}. This epigenetic model could serve to turn-on/off the DNA coding for the transcriptase reading. It could be applied to obtain a model of memory based in the natal language encryption readable on DNA.

During growing some of the first receptors expressed could be natal language and emotional experience. This could be used to assimilate receptors, within the first experiences required.

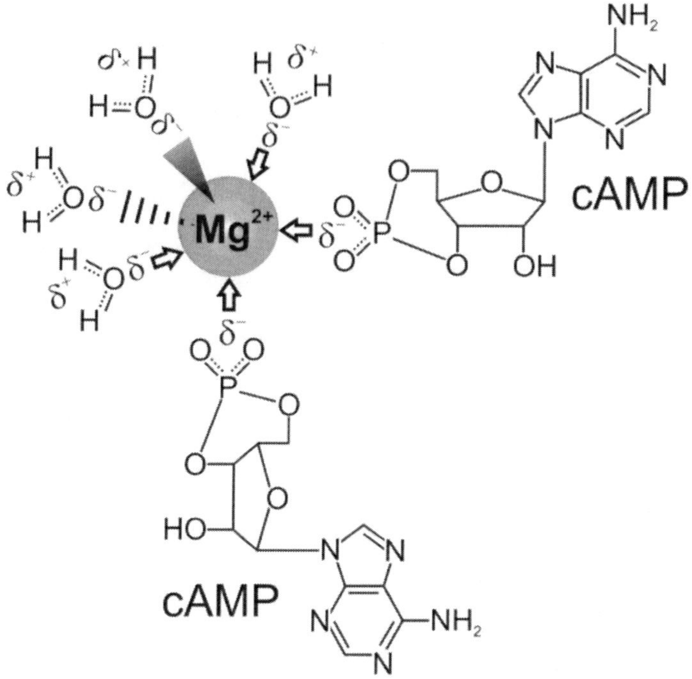

Figure 1. An Mg^{2+}-cAMP product, previously chelated by a protein R-groups, is released as an incomplete hydration shell. These promote an increase in the effective charge of the ion meriting the *nascent* denomination to Mg^{2+}. A following step could be the electrophilic attack on DNA by this *nascent* hydrated Mg^{2+}-cAMP enhanced simultaneously by coupling losses on the hydration shell.

The insertion of Mg^{2+}-cAMP opens the helix of the double-stranded DNA, to form a triple-stranded structure stabilized by pointing the purines and pyrimidines to the surface as showed in figure 3. This epigenetic mechanism provides coding for neuronal receptors.

The learned meaning could be adapted to emotional experience, for example: it would be required to the transcriptase to express the oxytocin (bonded to the membrane by Mg^{2+}) sequence for a primary event like forming the receptors required for bonding between mother and recently born child.

Other emotions like reward could be expressed by the sequence of the dopamine receptor. The CREB B-ZIP protein domain could respond to specific proteins which indicate a locus in DNA for the receptor to be expressed. Learning of the natal language is a long process accelerated when reaching encoding of the neuronal network.

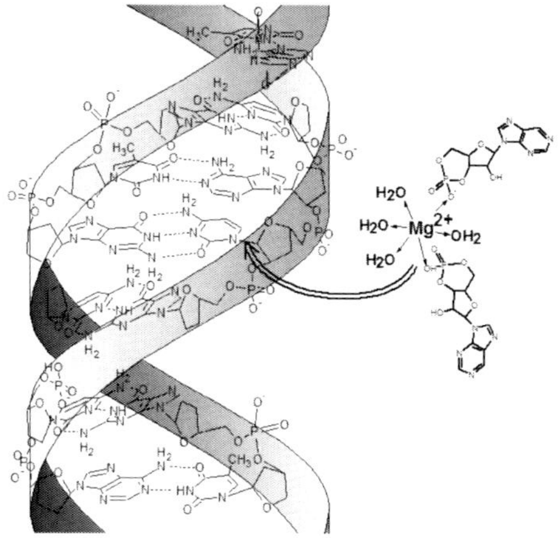

Figure 2. DNA-Mg-cAMP. The structure fitting function allows for DNA unzipping. cAMP/cGMP by binding to Mg2+ ion interacts with the negatively charged phosphate groups of a segment of DNA, wherein the base sequence of the two strands has a binary rotational symmetry about a center (palindromic 5'-TGACGTCA-3'). This displays the mechanism of transcriptional activation function called CREs (cAMP-responsive enhancers).

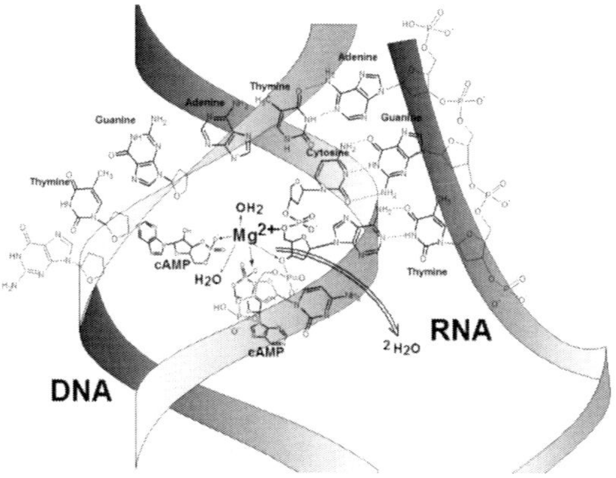

Figure 3. Crystallographic data has been used to find the fitting structure capable of playing the role of the CREB B-ZIP protein domain. In which a hexahydrated Mg^{2+} ion binds with additional cAMP for maintaining open the double-stranded DNA containing the consensus CRE sequence (5'-TGACGTCA-3').

However, this encoding at specific neurons could direct selecting the neuronal network to be turn-on.

cAMP transport in the absence of DNA and AC activity explains the role of red cells in the tissue regeneration.

When O_2 is released by Hb its affinity for Mg^{2+} is decreased, this became available for AC activation changing cellular cAMP levels. Uncontrolled process could trigger excessive cells duplication and cancer.

A negative charged ATP^{4-} or similar compound can turn the process reversible by subtracting the divalent metals.

cAMP DNA insertion could be adapted in expression of specific polypeptide for each receptor.

CONCLUSION

The search for models of the fitting structure between DNA and cAMP started by evaluate capability of Mg^{2+} and cAMP to modify control of DNA expression.

A unified mechanism for cAMP controlled DNA-reading shows a non-covalent hydration modifying activation of the coded DNA expression by the fitting-in of cAMP on DNA.

cAMP and cGMP studies on red cells revealed interactions [17] [18] [19]. The absence of DNA indicated that should be transported to regions were DNA expression was required.

Protein and H_2O are involved in energy expenditure during activation of protein synthesis turnover. In a protein the passage from its active to inactive states relates to the protein loss of H-bonds by a metabolic-dependent mechanism.

The release of water and metal by excess of ATP results on MgATP and the disappearance of free Mg^{2+}, which could inactivate AC and cAMP production [1] [2].

Attracting these groups resulted in the reorientation of the hydrophobic R-groups attracting between themselves.

The associated water through H-bonds leads to inactive architecture. In this context the H-bond loss from either hydrated state of proteins or DNA depends for turnover on entropy increase in the surrounding water [20]. This thermodynamics could characterize the homeostatic balance resulting from exhaled respiration saturated by vapor of water, eliminating entropy. The latter, do not contains H-bonds [21].

Assayed of cAMP and cGMP (Cyclic guanosine monophosphate) in red cells and cerebrospinal fluid (CSF) could be useful to obtain calibration tests, which physicians could relate to patients pathologic diagnosis.

Stress related diseases that through the fight-or-flight response mobilize metabolic reserves have a high consume phase that follows as an exhaustion phase. Oxytocin and serotonin adapt for modulated responses [22].

The testing of the cAMP and cGMP level should became a common practice in Hospitals because probably could contribute to early discover of neurodegenerative disorders. Subsequently, could allow for characterization of a disease progress and the probable outcome tendency.

Clinical could be expected that the assay of cAMP and cGMP in final phases of neurodegenerative diseases will show low concentration of this nucleotide. When as in Alzheimer in the brain appears empty areas, this could be related to the lack of regenerative protein capacity, because lack of cAMP turns inactive DNA. In Cancer development metabolic events leading to cell proliferation, may result from accumulation of cAMP and cGMP [23], showing uncontrolled transcription.

It could be expected that the assay of cAMP and cGMP in red cells and CSF could allow detecting in brain neurodegenerative diseases.

These characterizing these diseases by nucleotide value when well above the norm. Samples values correlating in a curve could allow the reading of results, in the detecting correlation curves. These results could characterize dysfunctions and the specific value when in deviation.

Similar effect could lead to the characterization of specific cancer [24], which could be probed by reagents testing for cAMP-cGMP in red cells and for neurodegeneration in CSF.

REFERENCES

[1] Brydon-Golz, S. and Bennun, A., Postsynthetic stabilized modification of adenylate cyclase by metabolites, *Biochemical Society Transactions,* 3, (1975), 721-724.

[2] Brydon-Golz, S., Ohanian, H. and Bennun, A., Effects of noradrenaline on the activation and the stability of brain adenylate cyclase, *Biochem. J.*, 166, (1977), 473-483.

[3] Bennun A. Book: Molecular Aspects of the Psychosomatic-Metabolic Axis and stress. Series: Neurology - Laboratory and Clinical Research Developments. Editorial: *Nova Science Publishers*, 2015. *ISBN: 978-1-63463-912-5.*

[4] [4] The New York Academy of Sciences. Learning from Cancer to Advance Drug Development for Neurodegeneration. Academy eBriefings. 2015. Available at: www.nyas.org/BDDGCancer-eB.

[5] Silva, A.J., Kogan, J. H., Frankland, P.W. and Kida, S. (1998) CREB and memory. *Annual Review of Neuroscience* 21, 127-148.

[6] Harris, R. and Bennun, A., Hormonal control of fat cells adenylate cyclase, *Molecular and Cellular Biochemistry*, 13, (1976), No. 3, 141-146.

[7] Harris, R.H., Cruz, R. and Bennun, A., The effect of hormones on metal and metal-ATP interactions with fat cell adenylate cyclase, Biosystems, 11, (1979), 29-46.

[8] Silva, A.J., Kogan, J. H., Frankland, P.W. and Kida, S. (1998) CREB and memory. *Annual Review of Neuroscience* 21, 127-148.

[9] [8] Davis, H. P. and Squire, L. R. (1984) Protein synthesis and memory: a review. Psychol. Bull. 96, 518–559.

[10] Mayr, B. and Montminy, M. (2001) Transcriptional regulation by the phosphorylation-dependent factor CREB. *Nat. Rev. Mol. Cell Biol.* 2(8), 599-609.

[11] Kandel, E.R. (2012) The molecular biology of memory: cAMP, PKA, CRE, CREB-1, CREB-2, and CPEB. *Mol. Brain* 5(1), 14.

[12] Kandel, E. R. (2001) The molecular biology of memory storage: a dialogue between genes and synapses. *Science* 294, 1030–1038.

[13] Bennun, A. and Blum, J.J. (1966) Properties of the induced acid phosphatase and of the constitutive acid phosphatase of Euglena. *Biochimica et Biophysica Acta*, 128, 106-123.

[14] Russo, D. (2008) The impact of kosmotropes and chaotropes on bulk and hydration shell water dynamics in a model peptide solution. *Chemical Physics* 345, 200–211.

[15] Bennun, A., A coupling mechanism to inter-relate regulatory with haem-haem interactions of haemoglobin, *Biomed. Biochim. Acta*, 46, (1987), No. 2/3, 314-319.

[16] Emma, J.E., Cervoni, P., Sulner, J.W. and Bennun, A., KCI-stimulated renin release, *Annals of the New York Academy of Sciences*, 463, (1986), 281-283.

[17] Bennun, A., Seidler, N. and De Bari, V.A., Divalent metals in the regulation of hemoglobin affinity for oxygen, *Annals of the New York Academy of Sciences*, 463, (1986), 76-79.

[18] DeBari, V. A. and Bennun, A. (1982). Cyclic GMP in the human erythrocyte. Intracellular levels and transport in normal subjects and chronic hemodialysis patients. *Clin. Biochem.,* 15, 219-221.

[19] Novembre, P.; Nicotra, J.; DeBari, V. A.; Needle, M. A. and Bennun, A. (1984). Erythrocyte transport of cyclic nucleotides. *Annals of the New York Academy of Sciences*, 435, 190-194.

[20]] DeBari, V. A.; Novak, N. A. and Bennun, A. (1984). Cyclic Nucleotide Metabolism in the Human Erythrocyte. *Clin. Physiol. Biochem.*, 2, 227-238.

[21] Bennun A. cAMP-Me2+-DNA Complex on Gene Induction and Signaling for Coupling the Environment Stimulus to Produce Variety and its Impact on Evolution. *Advances in Medicine and Biology*. Volume 98, Chapter10, Number xx, Pages xx-xx (2016).

[22] Bennun A. The coupling of thermodynamics with the organizational water-protein intra-dynamics driven by the H-bonds dissipative potential of water cluster. *Nova Publishers*. Submitted 07/04/2016.

[23] Bennun A. The Noradrenaline-Adrenaline-Axis of the Fight-or-Flight Exhibits Oxytocin and Serotonin Adaptive Responses. International Journal of Medical and Biological Frontiers. Volume 21, Issue 4, pages: 387-408 (2015).

[24] Fajardo, A. M.; Piazza, G. A.; Tinsley, H. N. (2014) The role of cyclic nucleotide signaling pathways in cancer: targets for prevention and treatment. *Cancers (Basel)*. 6(1):436-58.

[25] Miller, C. A.; Sweatt J. D. (2008) Covalent Modification of DNA Regulates Memory Formation. *Neuron*. 59(6), 1051.

In: Horizons in Cancer Research. Volume 63 ISBN: 978-1-53610-013-6
Editor: Hiroto S. Watanabe

Chapter 10

PROGNOSIS OF MALE BREAST CANCER

Patricia Tai[1], Derek Suderman[1] and Edward Yu[2]
[1]Department of Radiation Oncology, Allan Blair Cancer Center, Regina; University of Saskatchewan, Saskatchewan, Canada
[2]Department of Oncology and Division of Radiation Oncology, Western University, London, Ontario, Canada

ABSTRACT

Male breast cancer (MBC) comprises less than 1% of all cancers in men and less than 1% of all breast cancer in United States. In contrast to female breast cancer (FBC), male patients are generally older and have more advanced disease. MBC is rarely detected before age 30 and the mean age is 67 years. The advanced stage at presentation of MBC is thought to be related to thin breast parenchymal tissue in men. The tumors are often low or intermediate grade, with a higher percentage of ER-positive tumors. Patients with MBC routinely receive tamoxifen. All-cause mortality (ACM) is higher than FBC: for example in node-positive patients, all-cause mortality rate at 10-year was 67% in MBC versus 52% in FBC. There is a higher rate of distant recurrence for MBC. Factors such as advanced age, stage, visceral metastasis, triple-negative disease, androgen receptor, high grade, never married, smoking and low income at baseline are known to adversely affect outcome. The survival rates for MBC have lagged behind those for FBC. Prognosis may improve with more research on MBC in the future.

INTRODUCTION

Male breast cancer (MBC) is a rare disease worldwide. MBC accounts for approximately 1% of all breast cancers and less than 0.5% of all male cancer deaths in the United States [1]. The incidence seems to be increasing worldwide. The best estimate of incidence rate for MBC in all populations where data are available is 1/100,000 men. The highest reported incidence is 3.4/100,000 in Recife of Brazil, and the lowest in parts of Columbia, Singapore, Hungary, and Japan, at 0.1/100,000 [2].

The risk of developing MBC was positively associated with the following characteristics: never married, Ashkenazi Jewish ancestry, previous benign breast disease, gynecomastia, history of testicular pathology (cryptorchidism and/or orchitis), diabetes, prior liver disease, Klinefelter syndrome, family history of first-degree relatives with breast cancer and previous exposure to radiation [3].

In contrast to FBC, male patients are generally older and have more advanced disease. MBC is rarely detected before age 30 and the mean age is 67 years [4]. MBC differs from FBC in many respects, with higher incidence of BRCA1 (10%), lower incidence of BRCA2 (1%) and PIK3CA (20%) [5,6], more often estrogen receptor (ER)/ progesterone receptor (PR) positive, and less frequently positive for epidermal growth factor receptor-2 (HER2) [7]. Only 4% of MBC is triple negative [8]. The advanced stage at presentation of MBC is probably due to the thin breast parenchymal tissue in men [9] and cancer invades to the underlying muscles. Another reason for late presentation is due to the lack of awareness of breast cancer can rarely occur in men. Most breast tissue in men is located in the subareolar area, therefore, it typically presents as a painless, firm subareolar mass and the nipple soon becomes retracted. Because of the scanty breast tissue in men, lesions are close to the skin and tumor fixation to the pectoralis major and/or skin is more often observed. For early stage 0-IIIB breast cancer cases in a case-control series of 72 MBC and 72 FBC from Ottawa, mean disease-free survival was 127 months for women compared with 93 months for men ($p = 0.62$). Mean overall survival was 117 months for women compared with 124 months for men ($p = 0.35$) [10].

In patients 50 or older, MBC must be differentiated from various forms of senile breast hypertrophy associated with concomitant conditions or, more often, pharmacological treatments that interfere with hormonal metabolism.

Tumor pathology of MBC is more often low or intermediate grade, with a higher percentage of ER-positive tumors [5]. Invasive ductal carcinoma is the most common histopathologic subtype, accounting for 85% of all cases [8]. The remaining 15% of cases are ductal carcinoma in situ (DCIS) or papillary carcinomas. There are a few case reports of lobular carcinoma and lobular carcinoma in situ (LCIS) [11]. The rarity of lobular carcinoma and LCIS in male is thought to be due to the lack of acini and lobules in normal male breast tissue [11].

As in women, careful physical examination of the breast and the regional (axillary and supraclavicular) lymph nodes is essential in men presenting with a breast mass or a suspicious node. Because of late diagnosis, even small male breast cancers have a greater tendency to spread to the axillary lymph nodes. In addition to mammography, either core needle biopsy or fine-needle aspiration (FNA) for pathologic confirmation should be obtained. Although the efficacy of FNA in diagnosis of MBC is difficult to establish due to limited case series reported in the literature, adequate tissue sampling is critical for establishing the diagnosis and performing ER, PR, and HER2 receptor analysis.

PROGNOSTIC FACTORS

Similar to FBC, stage, tumor size, and axillary lymph node status appear to be the most important factors influencing outcomes. MBC is associated with higher all-cause mortality. In one series of node-positive breast cancer patients, all-cause mortality at 10-year was 67% for men versus 52% for women.4 MBC has a higher rate of distant disease recurrence [12]. Poor prognostic factors include advanced age, histologic grade or stage [13], visceral metastasis, triple-negative disease [14], androgen receptor positivity [15], high histological grade, Ki-67 > 20% [16], never married [17], smokers [18], under-treatment, comorbidities, payer's status [19], African American[20], and low income at baseline. This chapter will also discuss other potential prognostic factors such as resection margin, use of hormonal therapy, chemotherapy and radiation therapy (RT).

Staging

Both male and female breast cancers are staged according to the American Joint Committee on Cancer (AJCC) staging system [21] (Table 1). Although the prognosis in men has often been cited as similar to stage-matched female patients, men tend to fare worse overall, partly due to late presentation and consequently with more advanced disease [22] (Table 2).

In one analysis from Serbia, 44% of MBC presented with stage I or II disease, 46.4% stage III, and 9.5% stage IV [23]. One-fifth of all patients had tumors measuring $\leq$2 cm, and 14.3% were larger than 5 cm. Lymph node metastases were documented in 40.4% of patients, of which 47% relapsed. Overall survival for all patients at five and ten years was 55.0% and 43.9%, respectively.

Table 1. Breast cancer staging

Primary tumor (T)

Tx Primary tumor cannot be assessed

T0 No evidence of primary tumor

Tis Carcinoma in situ

T1 Tumor 20 mm or less in greatest dimension

T1mi </= 1 mm

T1a > 1 mm but <= 5 mm

T1b > 5 mm but <= 10 mm

T1c > 10 mm but <= 20 mm

T2 Tumor more than 2 cm but not more than 5 cm in greatest dimension

T3 Tumor more than 5 cm in greatest dimension

T4 Tumor with direct extension to the chest wall and/or to the skin

T4a Extension to the chest wall, not including only pectoralis muscle adherence/invasion

T4b Ulceration and/or ipsilateral satellite nodules and/or edema (including peau d'orange) of the skin, which do not meet the criteria for inflammatory carcinoma

T4c Both T4a and T4b

T4d Inflammatory carcinoma

Regional lymph node (N)

Clinical

Nx Regional lymph nodes cannot be assessed

N0 No regional lymph node metastasis
N1 Metastases to movable ipsilateral level I, II *axillary lymph node(s)*
N2
N2a Metastases to ipsilateral level I, II *axillary lymph node* fixed to one another (matted) or other structures
N2b Metastases in *clinically detected internal mammary* nodes in the absence of level I, II axillary node metastases
N3
N3a Metastases in ipsilateral *infraclavicular* node(s)
N3b Metastases in *ipsilateral internal mammary node(s) and axillary* node(s)
N3c Metastases in *ipsilateral supraclavicular* node(s)

Pathologic (pN)
pNx Regional lymph nodes cannot be assessed
pN0 No regional lymph node metastasis histologically. Isolated tumor cell clusters (ITC, i) are defined as small clusters of cells *not greater than 0.2 mm*, or single tumor cells, or a cluster of fewer than 200 cells in a single histologic cross-section. ITCs may be detected by routine histology (hematoxylin and eosin stain, H&E) or by immunohistochemical (IHC) methods
pN0(i-) Negative IHC
pN0(i+) ITC not greater than 0.2 mm detected by H&E or IHC
pN0(mol-) negative molecular findings by reverse transcriptase/polymerase chain reaction (RT-PCR)
pN0(mol+) positive molecular findings by RT-PCR but not detected by histology or IHC
pN1
pN1mi Micrometastases (> 0.2 mm and/or >200 cells but *none > 2 mm*)
pN1a Metastases in *1-3 axillary* lymph nodes, at least one metastasis > 2 mm
pN1b Metastases in *internal mammary* nodes with micrometastases or macrometastases detected by sentinel lymph node biopsy (SLNB) but not clinically detected
pN1c Metastases in *1-3 axillary lymph nodes and in internal mammary* nodes with micrometastases or macrometastases detected by SLNB but not clinically detected
pN2

pN2a Metastases in *4-9 axillary* lymph nodes, at least one metastasis > 2 mm

pN2b Metastases in *clinically detected internal mammary* nodes in the absence of axillary node metastases

pN3

pN3a Metastases in *10 or more axillary* lymph nodes, at least one metastasis > 2 mm; or metastases to the *infraclavicular* (level III axillary lymph) nodes

pN3b Metastases in clinically detected *ipsilateral internal mammary nodes in the presence of one or more positive axillary* node metastases; or >*3 axillary lymph nodes and in internal mammary* nodes with micrometastases or macrometastases detected by SLNB but not clinically detected

pN3c Metastases in *ipsilateral supraclavicular* (level III axillary lymph) nodes

Distant metastasis (M)

M0 No clinical or radiographic evidence of distant metastases

cM0(i+)No clinical or radiographic evidence of distant metastases, but deposits of molecularly or microscopically detected tumor cells in circulating blood, bone marrow or other nonregional nodal tissue that are *not larger than 0.2 mm* in a patient without symptoms or signs of metastases

M1 Distant detectable metastasis as determined by classic clinical and radiographic means and/or histologically proven larger than 0.2 mm

Stage grouping

Stage 0	Tis N0 M0	
Stage IA	T1 N0 M0	
Stage IB	T0-1 N1mi M0	
Stage IIA	T0-1 N1 M0 or	T2 N0 M0
Stage IIB	T2 N1 M0 or	T3 N0 M0
Stage IIIA	T0-2 N2 M0 or	T3 N1-2 M0
Stage IIIB	T4 N0-2 M0	
Stage IIIC	anyT N3 M0	
Stage IV	anyT anyN M1	

Table 2. Male breast cancer outcome from Surveillance Epidemiology and End Results (SEER) database of the United States treated with surgery and radiotherapy (simplified from reference 23)

Stage	5 year	10 year
Overall survival (%)		
I	88%	80%
II	75%	50%
III	50%	30%
IV	30%	10%
Cause-specific survival (%)		
I	98%	90%
II	90%	75%
III	60%	50%
IV	40%	15%

Genetic Factors

BRCA2 MBC tends to be higher grade [24]. Tamoxifen is converted to active form by the polymorphic CYP2D6 enzyme. Patients with the A allele in a homozygous or heterozygous form are poor tamoxifen metabolizers. Genotyping from blood or tumor found that being a poor metabolizer had a significantly higher recurrence rate and lower survival [25]. Poorer survival outcome is significantly associated with whole arm copy number gains of 17q, in which the NEUROD2 gene is located [26].

Pathologic Factors

The presence of any of basal or mesenchymal markers correlated with a more advanced tumor stage [27]. Moreover, tumors without vimentin expression were characterised by lower MIB-1 LI and were more frequently EGFR immuno-negative. Hormone receptor negativity, vimentin immuno-positivity and high MIB-1 LI are significant independent indicators of poor OS and DFS for MBC patients ($p < 0.05$). ER and PR expression was positive in 66.7-95% (in different series) and 58.3%, respectively. Tumors were HER2 positive in 14.3% of patients [23].

Surgical Resection Margin

For localized MBC, the current procedure of choice is total mastectomy with sentinel node (SLN) biopsy. Although breast conservation therapy with lumpectomy followed by breast irradiation has been shown to have equivalent outcomes compared to mastectomy in women with early stage breast cancer, breast conservation therapy is generally not considered as an option for men because the tumor is almost always in the central quadrant, which necessitates removal of the nipple areola, effectively warranting removal of the majority of the breast tissue.

A PubMed search does not reveal any publication regarding the significance of margin status for MBC. Our own multivariate analysis did not show it to be an independent prognostic factor [28].

Use of Adjuvant Endocrine Therapy

MBC are often positive for ER and PR. Previous data indicate improvements in disease-free and overall survival in MBC patients given hormonal treatments such as diethylstilbestrol, medroxyprogesterone, luteinizing hormone- releasing hormone (LHRH) agonist and/or orchiectomy, in comparison with historical controls. Tamoxifen remains the drug of choice for adjuvant treatment, as aromatase inhibitors are less effective in men [5]. Tamoxifen is routinely recommended for 5 years. One study reported an improved 5-year actuarial survival (61% vs 44%) and disease-free survival (55% vs 28%) in 39 patients who received tamoxifen compared with historical controls [29,30]. Tamoxifen is generally well tolerated. The most common side effects in men include decreased libido, weight gain, hot flashes, mood alteration and depression. Data in the adjuvant setting on the use of fulvestrant in MBC is limited.

Use of Adjuvant Chemotherapy

Because of the low incidence, recommendations for adjuvant systemic therapy for MBC are derived from clinical trials for FBC. In view of the toxicity of chemotherapy and the fact that over 30% of MBC patients are 70 or older [31], adjuvant chemotherapy should be strongly considered in men with receptor-negative disease and/or high risk of recurrence.

In an NCI study of 24 MBC patients with node-positive stage II disease treated with adjuvant cyclophosphamide, methotrexate, and 5-fluorouracil (CMF), 5-year survival was 80% and median survival was 98 months, significantly better than historical controls [32]. A study from MD Anderson Cancer Center involving node-positive MBC treated with CMF, with 20 years follow up, reported overall survival rates at 5, 10, and 20 years of 85%, 65%, and 42% respectively [33]. These data suggest that for selected node positive MBC, adjuvant chemotherapy is appropriate and can be beneficial.

Use of Adjuvant Radiation Therapy

There is no prospective randomized clinical trial available that evaluates the role of adjuvant radiation therapy in MBC. Although the technical aspects of radiation therapy varied over time and between series making assessment of the clinical impact of post-mastectomy radiation therapy (PMRT) difficult, there are several series which report a benefit of PMRT [34,35]. It reduced locoregional recurrence for MBC, but had no impact on overall survival [36,37]. In our study of 75 MBC patients treated with PMRT, the local relapse rate was 4% compared with 24% for those receiving surgery alone [38]. Locoregional control was greater in high risk patients (close resection margin, positive node and advance stage). Other studies have suggested that the same indications for PMRT that apply to women should be used in men [39]. Studies of women who received PMRT showing a survival advantage [40,41]. may be applicable for MBC patients with similar stage.

Use of Systemic Therapy in Metastatic Disease

A great majority of breast cancers in men are endocrine responsive, and in fact, orchiectomy used to be the standard of care for treatment of metastatic MBC, together with other aggressive surgical procedures such as hypophysectomy and adrenalectomy as primary treatment modalities.

Orchiectomy was reported to have response rates between 32% and 67%, with a median survival of 56 months in responding patients compared to 38 months in non-responding patients [42]. Castration also increases the probability of response to second-line ablative treatment, and some patients who failed orchiectomy responded to adrenalectomy or other endocrine treatment such as tamoxifen [43]. Aggressive surgical interventions are rarely used today, and medication is an attractive alternative as it avoids surgical morbidity and mortality, is reversible and is psychologically more acceptable to most men.

Tamoxifen is considered to be the first line treatment for metastatic male breast cancer at present, with overall response rates of 49% reported [44]. However, there is no prospective randomized trial to more robustly evaluate the response rates and toxicity of tamoxifen in men.

The new selective aromatase inhibitors (anastrozole, letrozole, and exemestane) are very active and widely used agents for treatment of advanced disease in postmenpausal women with hormone receptor-positive breast cancer. Experience with their use in MBC is limited [45,46]. A study comparing the monotherapy of aromatase inhibitor or cyproterone acetate versus combination with gonadotropin-releasing hormone analogue for metastatic MBC showed the 2-year survival rates were 44% vs 65% (P = 0.05) [47].

Fulvestrant, a 7–alkylamide derivative of estradiol, is an estrogen antagonist [48] that competitively binds to and degrades estrogen receptors in human breast cancer tissue. It has been demonstrated to be effective in postmenopausal women with metastatic breast cancer. For metastatic MBC, fulvestrant is used in tamoxifen-resistant patients [49,50].

For androgen receptor positive MBC, the overall survival and time to progression are shorter than those without androgen receptors, and tamoxifen seems to be less helpful in those patients [51]. Antiandrogens and cyproterone acetate have been tried with some success [52].

Systemic chemotherapy is usually considered a second-line therapy in metastatic MBC. Chemotherapy can provide significant palliation after hormonal therapy has failed, or in those with receptor-negative disease, or life-threatening visceral disease. The overall response rate for all chemotherapy regimens in men has been estimated at 40% [53].

Data for other chemotherapy agents such as taxanes [54], capecitabine, vinorebine or gemcitabine in men is limited. Similarly, there is little information currently available on the benefits of trastuzumab in the rare MBC cases which are HER2-positive.

In summary, for patients with metastatic disease, chemotherapy should be recommended for hormone receptor-negative, or rapidly progressing disease. Tamoxifen should be considered for patients with indolent hormone receptor-positive disease. Median survival from occurrence of metastasis was 32 months in a German series of 41 treated MBC.

References

[1] http://www.cancer.gov/search/results.

[2] Giordano SH, Perkin GH, BroglioK, et al. Adjuvant systemic therapy for male breast cancer. *Cancer* 2005;104(11): 2359-64.

[3] Brinton LA, Cook MB, McCormack V, et al. Anthropometric and hormonal risk factors for male breast cancer: male breast cancer pooling project results. *J. Natl. Cancer Inst.* 2014;106(3): djt465.

[4] Yu E, Stitt L, Vujovic O, Joseph K, et al. Prognostic factors for male breast cancer, are they similar to their female counterparts? *Anticancer. Research* 2013;33: 2227-32.

[5] Fentiman IS. Male breast cancer is not congruent with the female disease. *Crit. Rev. Oncol. Hematol.* 2016 Feb 27. pii: S1040-8428(16)30041-5. [Epub ahead of print].

[6] Piscuoglio S, Ng CK, Murray MP, et al. The Genomic Landscape of Male Breast Cancers. *Clin. Cancer Res.* 2016 Mar 9. pii: clincanres.2840.2015. [Epub ahead of print].

[7] Yu XF, Yang HJ, Yu Y, et al. A prognostic analysis of male breast cancer (MBC) compared with post-menopausal female breast cancer (FBC). *PLoS One.* 2015;10(8): e0136670.

[8] Aggarwal A, Liu ML, Krasnow SH. Breast cancer in male veteran population: an analysis from VA cancer registry. *J. Community Support Oncol.* 2014;12(8): 293-7.

[9] Jamy O(1), Rafiq A, Laghari A, et al. Male breast cancer: a 24 year experience of a tertiary care hospital in Pakistan. *Asian Pac. J. Cancer Prev.* 2015;16(4): 1559-63.

[10] Rushton M, Kwong A, Visram H, et al. Treatment outcomes for male breast cancer: a single-centre retrospective case-control study. *Curr. Oncol.* 2014;21(3): e400-7.

[11] Zahir MN, Minhas K, Shabbir-Moosajee M. Pleomorphic lobular carcinoma of the male breast with axillary lymph node involvement: a case report and review of literature. *BMC Clin. Pathol.* 2014 Apr 27;14: 16.

[12] Serarslan A(1), Gursel B, Okumus NO, et al. Male Breast Cancer: 20 Years Experience of a Tertiary Hospital from the Middle Black Sea Region of Turkey. *Asian Pac. J. Cancer Prev.* 2015;16(15): 6673-9.

[13] Oger AS, Boukerrou M, Cutuli B, et al. Male breast cancer: prognostic factors, diagnosis and treatment: a multi-institutional survey of 95 cases. *Gynecol. Obstet. Fertil.* 2015;43(4): 290-6.

[14] Leone JP, Leone J, Zwenger AO, et al. Prognostic significance of tumor subtypes in male breast cancer: a population-based study. *Breast Cancer Res. Treat.* 2015;152(3):601-9.

[15] Di Lauro L, Barba M, Pizzuti L, et al. Androgen receptor and antiandrogen therapy in male breast cancer. *Cancer Lett.* 2015;368(1): 20-5.

[16] Masci G, Caruso M, Caruso F, et al. Clinicopathological and immunohistochemical characteristics in male breast cancer: a retrospective case series. *Oncologist.* 2015;20(6): 586-92.

[17] O'Brien B, Koru-Sengul T, Miao F, et al. Disparities in Overall Survival for Male Breast Cancer Patients in the State of Florida (1996-2007). *Clin. Breast Cancer.* 2015;15(4): e177-87.

[18] Padron-Monedero A, Koru-Sengul T, Tannenbaum SL, et al. Smoking and survival in male breast cancer patients. *Breast Cancer Res. Treat.* 2015;153(3): 679-87.

[19] Shi R, Taylor H, Liu L, et al. Private Payer's Status Improves Male Breast Cancer Survival. *Breast J.* 2016;22(1): 101-4.

[20] Shin JY, Kachnic LA, Hirsch AE. The impact of race in male breast cancer treatment and outcome in the United States: a population-based analysis of 4,279 patients. *Int. J. Breast Cancer.* 2014;2014: 685842.

[21] https://www.nccn.org/professionals/physician_gls/pdf/breast.pdf.

[22] Madden NA, Macdonald OK, Call JA, et al. Radiotherapy and male breast cancer: a population-based registry analysis. *Am. J. Clin. Oncol.* 2014 Apr 28.

[23] Sipetic-Grujicic SB, Murtezani ZH, Neskovic-Konstatinovic ZB, et al. Multivariate analysis of prognostic factors in male breast cancer in Serbia. *Asian Pac. J. Cancer Prev.* 2014;15(7): 3233-8.

[24] Silvestri V, Barrowdale D, Mulligan AM, et al. Male breast cancer in BRCA1 and BRCA2 mutation carriers: pathology data from the Consortium of Investigators of Modifiers of BRCA1/2. *Breast Cancer Res.* 2016;18(1): 15.

[25] Abreu MH, Gomes M, Menezes F, et al. CYP2D6*4 polymorphism: A new marker of response to hormonotherapy in male breast cancer? *Breast.* 2015;24(4): 481-6.

[26] Lacle MM, Moelans CB, Kornegoor R, et al. Chromosome 17 copy number changes in male breast cancer. *Cell Oncol. (Dordr).* 2015;38(3): 237-45.
[27] Sas-Korczynska B, Niemiec J, Harazin-Lechowska A, et al. The biological markers and results of treatment in male breast cancer patients. The Cracow experience. *Neoplasma.* 2014;61(3): 331-9.
[28] Yu E, Stitt L, Vujovic O, et al. Male breast cancer prognostic factors versus female counterparts with propensity scores and matched-pair analysis. *Cureus* 2015;7(10): e355.
[29] Ribeiro G, Swindell R. Adjuvant tamoxifen for male breast cancer. *Br. J. Cancer.* 1992;65(2): 252-4.
[30] Early Breast Cancer Trialists Collaborative Group: Tamoxifen for early breast cancer: an overview of randomized trials. *Lancet* 1998;351: 1451-67.
[31] Crichlow RW. Carcinoma of the male breast. *Surg gynecol obstet.* 1972;134: 11011-9.
[32] Bagley CS, Wesley MN, Young RC, et al. Adjuvant chemotherapy in males with cancer of the breast. *Am. J. Clin. Oncol.* 1987;10(1): 55-60.
[33] Walshe JM, Berman AW, Vatas U, et al. A prospective study of adjuvant CMF in male with node positive breast cancer :20-year follow –up. *Breast Cancer Res Treat.* 2007;103(2):177-83.
[34] Erlichman C, Murphy KC, Elhakim T. Male breast cancer: a 13 year review of 89 patients. *J. Clin. Oncol.* 1984;(2(8): 903-9.
[35] Chung HC,Koh EH, Roth JK, et al, Male breast cancer- a 20 year review of 16 cases at Yonsei University. *Yonsei Med. J.* 1990;31: 242-50.
[36] Cutuli B, Lacroze M, Dilhuydy JM, et al. Male breast cancer: Results of the treatment and prognostic factors in 397 cases. *Euro J. cancer.* 1995;31A; 1960-4.
[37] Willsher PC, leach IH, Ellis IO, et al. A comparison outcome of male breast cancer with female breast cancer. *Am. J. Surg.* 1997;172: 185-8.
[38] Yu E, Suzuki H, Younus J, et al. Impact of post mastectomy radiation therapy on male breast cancer patients - a case series. *Int. J. Radiat. Oncol. Biol. Phys.* 2012;82: 696-700.
[39] Vindo SK , Pendlebury SC. Carcinoma of the male breast: A review of adjuvant therapy. *Australas Radiol.* 1999;43: 69-72.
[40] Overgaard m, Hansen PS, Overgaard J, et al. Postoperative radiotherapy in high-risk premenopausal women with breast cancer who receive adjuvant chemotherapy. Danish Breast Cancer Cooperative group 82b trial. *N. Eng. J. Med.* 1997;337(14): 949-55.

[41] EBCTCG (Early Breast Cancer Trialists' Collaborative Group), McGale P, Taylor C, et al. Effect of radiotherapy after mastectomy and axillary surgery on 10-year recurrence and 20-year breast cancer mortality: meta-analysis of individual patient data for 8135 women in 22 randomised trials. *Lancet.* 2014;383(9935): 2127-35.
[42] Donegan WL, Redlich PN. Breast cancer in men. *Surg Clin North Am.* 1996;76(2):343-63.
[43] Becher R, hoffken K, Pape H, et al. Tamoxofen treatment before orchiectomy in advanced breast cancer in men. *N. Engl. J. Med.* 1981;305: 169-70.
[44] Nahleh ZA. Hormone therapy for male breast cancer: a different approach for a different disease. *Cancer Treat. Rev.* 2006;32: 101-5.
[45] Kuba S, Ishida M, Oikawa M, et al. Aromatase inhibitors with or without luteinizing hormone-releasing hormone agonist for metastatic male breast cancer: report of four cases and review of the literature. *Breast Cancer.* 2016 Feb 15. [Epub ahead of print].
[46] Maugeri-Saccà M, Barba M, Vici P, et al. Aromatase inhibitors for metastatic male breast cancer: molecular, endocrine, and clinical considerations. *Breast Cancer Res. Treat.* 2014;147(2): 227-35.
[47] Di Lauro L, Pizzuti L, Barba MJ, et al. Role of gonadotropin-releasing hormone analogues in metastatic male breast cancer: results from a pooled analysis. *Hematol Oncol.* 2015;8:53.
[48] Osborne CK, Corondo-Heinsohn EB, Hilsenbeck SG, et al. Comparison of the effects of a pure steroidal antiestrogen with those of tamoxifen in a model of human breast cancer. *J. Natl. Cancer Inst.* 1995;87: 746-50.
[49] Agrawal A, Cheung KI, Robertson JF. Fulvestrant in advanced male breast cancer. *Breast Cancer Res.Treat.* 2007; 101: 123.
[50] Zagouri F, Sergentanis TN, Chrysikos D, et al. Fulvestrant and male breast cancer: a pooled analysis. *Breast Cancer Res. Treat.* 2015;149(1): 269-75.
[51] Wenhui Z, Shuo L, Dabei T, et al. Androgen receptor expression in male breast cancer predicts inferior outcome and poor response to tamoxifen treatment. *Eur. J. Endocrinol.* 2014;171(4): 527-33.
[52] Di Lauro L(1), Vici P, Barba M, et al. Antiandrogen therapy in metastatic male breast cancer: results from an updated analysis in an expanded case series. *Breast Cancer Res Treat.* 2014;148(1): 73-80.
[53] Kraybill WG, Kaufman R, Kinne D. Treatment of advanced male breast cancer. *Cancer* 1981;47: 2185-9.

[54] Huang DP, Ye XH, Jin C. Successful use of bevacizumb and paclitaxel in a male breast cancer with liver metastases. *Int. J. Clin. Exp. Med.* 2014;7(9): 3076-9.

INDEX

A

B

C

D

E

F

G

H

I

J

K

L

M

N

O

P

S

T

U

V

W

X

Y

Z